Hospital-acquired Infection

The authors would like to dedicate this book to Barry Collins who died in 1989. He was an author of the first two editions and was particularly well known for his work on the role of the environment in the spread of infection, decontamination of equipment and infection problems in the domestic and catering fields.

Hospital-acquired infection

Principles and prevention

Third edition

G A J Ayliffe MD, FRCPath

Emeritus Professor of Medical Microbiology, University of Birmingham;
Honorary Consultant, formerly Director, Hospital Infection Research Laboratory,
City Hospital NHS Trust, Birmingham, UK

J R Babb FIBMS

Laboratory Manager, Hospital Infection Research Laboratory, City Hospital
NHS Trust, Birmingham, UK

Lynda J Taylor MBA, RGN, RM

Infection Control Unit, Laboratory of Hospital Infection, Central Public Health
Laboratory, Colindale, London, UK

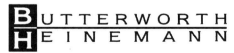

OXFORD AUCKLAND BOSTON JOHANNESBURG MELBOURNE NEW DELHI

Butterworth-Heinemann
Linacre House, Jordan Hill, Oxford OX2 8DP
225 Wildwood Avenue, Woburn, MA 01801-2041
A division of Reed Educational and Professional Publishing Ltd

℞   A member of the Reed Elsevier plc group

First published 1982
Reprinted 1983
Second edition 1990
Reprinted 1991, 1993
Third edition 1999

British Library Cataloguing in Publication Data
A catalogue record for this book is available from the British Library

Library of Congress Cataloguing in Publication Data
A catalogue record for this book is available from the Library of Congress

ISBN 0 7506 2105 2

Typeset by Latimer Trend & Company Ltd, Plymouth
Printed and bound by MPG Books Ltd, Bodmin, Cornwall

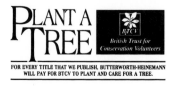

Contents

Foreword

The control of infection in hospitals has been greatly improved and its principles more widely understood in recent years, thanks to a number of important developments; these include much research by microbiologists and clinicians, effective surveillance of infection through the appointment of infection control teams, officers and nurses, the introduction of central sterile supply, improved communication to all of those involved in patient care through training programmes, conferences and publications such as this book. Today no surgeon would claim, as some did in the not-so-distant past, that patients in their wards do not become infected. Methods used in the control of infection are today chosen on the basis of evidence that they are effective, not time-honoured but untested rituals, such as many were until recent times.

In spite of these improvements the incidence of hospital infection is about as high today as it has been for many years. This is not entirely surprising, for seriously ill patients are often highly susceptible to infection and the methods of controlling infection in such cases are very poor. The factors involved in hospital-acquired infection are complex; they include acquisition by patients of many kinds of micro-organisms varying in virulence and distribution, and the exposure of patients with widely varying susceptibility to these micro-organisms. Much infection is sporadic, but outbreaks occur from time to time, due either to the appearance of exceptionally virulent organisms in the hospital or to the exceptional presence of bacteria on items used in surgery which should be sterile. There have been fluctuations in the severity and prevalence of some infections, and some new kinds of infection have emerged. Antibiotics, which transformed the prospects for patients with bacterial infection in the second half of this century, lost some of their usefulness because of the emergence and spread of antibiotic resistant strains, including those with multiple resistance and transferable resistance; these are increasing hazards today. The use of antibiotics leads to the selection and spread of resistant bacteria; all inessential use of antibiotics in hospital must therefore be avoided. Antibiotic therapy can be seen as a 'battle' between bacterial genes, which cannot avoid obeying their genetic codes, and human wits, which invent but usually fail to obey their codes of practice. We need all the ingenuity we can muster in our attempts to outwit such wily opponents. Those who take up infection control duties will find that

Professor Ayliffe and his co-authors provide in this book a valuable guide to a subject that involves the application of many disciplines. It presents in straightforward terms a wide range of microbiological information, much of it based on the authors' personal observations and research through many years.

E. J. L. Lowbury DM, DSC, FRCPath

Preface

Hospital-acquired infection remains a worldwide problem. In recent national prevalence surveys of hospital infection in the UK, and in other developed countries, the acquired infection rate was still about 10%. Infections occurred mainly in patients with unavoidable risk factors, e.g. the elderly, the immunocompromised, those with invasive devices or following surgery. Surveillance is an important component of an infection control programme and the measurement of infecton rates would seem to be an appropriate index of the efficacy of control procedures. However, reliable comparisons of infection rates between hospitals are rarely possible owing to the number of variable risk factors and the difficulties of compensating for them. In addition, rapid discharge from hospital, especially following minimal access surgery, means that hospital-acquired infection will often first become manifest in the community.

The increasing cost of preventing infection has led to a requirement for proven cost-effective measures, based on risk assessment and, where possible, on evidence-based guidelines. The mental state and physical comfort of infected patients are now more frequently considered when making infection control decisions, e.g. on the isolation of elderly patients in single rooms.

New or re-emerging infections continue to cause problems. These include those with highly antibiotic-resistant enterococci, Gram-negative bacilli, *Staphylococcus aureus, Clostridium difficile* and *Mycobacterium tuberculosis*. Methicillin-resistant *Staph. aureus* is spreading in hospitals around the world, often despite maximum efforts to control it.

Bloodborne viral infections, e.g. hepatitis B and C and HIV, still cause anxiety to hospital staff and, although transmission is rare either to staff or other patients, methods designed to prevent their spread are playing a prominant role in day-to-day infection control practices.

The increase in the use of expensive heat-labile equipment, e.g. flexible endoscopies, requires a high-quality system for decontamination. Nevertheless, basic infection control procedures, such as handwashing, are not necessarily expensive and have changed very little; the main problem is with policy compliance. These procedures not only require initial education of medical and nursing staff, but follow-up training and regular audit. Audit should concentrate on procedures likely to influence the acquisition of infection and not on rituals, such as environmental sampling.

It is hoped that this book will provide health care staff with sufficient knowledge to understand the mechanisms of transmission of infection, contributing factors and methods of prevention. It does not include detailed guidelines or procedures, but contains information on the underlying basis of these and will help staff to make their own decisions. It deals with administration of infection control, basic properties of relevant micro-organisms, risk factors, nursing procedures and methods of decontamination. It also gives advice on catering and laundry hygiene, and disposal of clinical waste. The rational use of antibiotics is not discussed in detail, but is well covered in other books. The references have been updated, but the reader is referred to other, larger, textbooks and journals for more complete lists of references.

The book is based mainly on lectures given by the authors. Although it is primarily an introduction for infection control practitioners, much of the information should also be useful to nurse teachers, trainee surgeons, trainee microbiologists and Control of Communicable Disease Consultants, SSD managers, domestic supervisors, engineers and pharmacists. It should also prove useful to the manufacturers of infection-control-related products and those providing contractual services to hospitals.

1

Administrative aspects of infection control

Introduction

In most countries, 5–10% of patients in hospital at any one time have acquired an infection. The recent National Prevalence Survey in the UK and Ireland (1993–1994) showed a prevalence of hospital-acquired infection of 9.0% (range 2–29%) (Emmerson and Ayliffe, 1996). These infections were mainly of the urinary tract (23%), surgical wounds (10.7%), the lower respiratory tract (22.9%) and the skin (9.6%) (Table 1.1). The overall prevalence was similar to the previous survey in 1980, i.e 9.2%, but there were differences in the two surveys, both in the types of patient and the number of hospitals involved. The calculation of risk factors may also show further differences in the patient populations. There was an apparent fall in surgical wound infections from 18.9% in 1980 to 10.7%, but this may have been due to more postoperative infections emerging in the community following an increase in day surgery and reduced hospital stay. The WHO survey showed a similar range of infections with a wide variation between hospitals (Mayon White *et al.*, 1988). Children under 1 year showed a higher rate (prevalence 13.5%) with a predominance of respiratory, gastrointestinal

Table 1.1 Prevalence of hospital-acquired infection						
	Overall (%)	Urinary tract (%)	Surgical wounds (%)	Lower respiratory tract (%)	Skin (%)	Other (%)
UK (1)–1980 45 hospitals 18 163 patients	9.2	2.8	1.7	1.5	1.2	2.0
WHO–1983–5 47 hospitals (14 countries) 28 861 patients	8.4 (3–21)	0.3–4.7	0.3–3.1	1.1–4.1	0.5–3.2	0.3–2.4
UK (2)–1994 153 hospitals 37 000 patients	9.0	2.4	1.1	2.4	1.0	2.1

Table 1.2   Organisms causing hospital-acquired infection (Prevalence Survey, UK and Ireland, 1994)

Organism	Percentage of isolates from infections
Escherichia coli	20.1
Staphylococcus aureus	14.7
Methicillin-resistant *Staph. aureus*	5.0
Coagulase-negative staphylococci	7.7
Enterococci	7.0
Pseudomonas aeruginosa	6.7
Misc. Gram-negative bacilli, *Klebsiella, Proteus,* } *Enterobacter, Acinetobacter* spp.	8.0
Streptococcus pneumoniae	1.2

and skin infections. An incidence study carried out in 19 hospitals in the UK over 1 year showed a mean infection rate of 2.7 per 100 patient-episodes in 80 752 patients (Glynn *et al.*, 1997). The study included the urinary tract (1.6 per 100 patient-episodes), the lower respiratory tract (0.74 per 100 patient-episodes) and bloodstream infections (0.30 per 100 patient-episodes), but not surgical wounds. Where a device was used, the infection rate was 7.2 per 100 patient-episodes, confirming the importance of invasive devices as risk factors for infection.

The overall results of reports of surveys around the world indicate that hospital infection is still a major problem in all countries. However, many of these infections are minor and deaths directly due to acquired infection are infrequent, although these infections are often a contributory factor. Infection rates are highest in special units such as intensive care, burns, special care baby units and units for immunosuppressed patients.

Infection is mainly associated with factors which increase the risks of acquiring infection, e.g. greater susceptibility of the patient and an increase in the number of invasive procedures. Neonates, the elderly and the immunocompromised are particularly susceptible. Urinary infections are usually associated with urethral catheterization, lower respiratory infections with endotracheal intubation and mechanical ventilation, and bacteraemias are often associated with intravascular catherization (Glynn *et al.*, 1997).

The predominant organisms causing infection are shown in Table 1.2. Infections caused by coagulase-negative staphylococci, vancomycin-resistant enterococci (VRE) and methicillin-resistant *Staphylococcus aureus* (MRSA) have increased in recent years. Most hospital-acquired infections are endogenous in origin, i.e acquired from the patient's own normal flora of the skin, respiratory tract or gastrointestinal tract. Exogenous infections (cross-infection) are mainly acquired from infected patients or less frequently from healthy carriers or medical equipment. Transmission is mainly on the hands of staff. The dry inanimate environment is rarely a source, but may be a reservoir or route of spread. Although outbreaks of clinical infection usually represent a relatively small proportion of the total hospital-acquired infection, they may involve hospital infection control staff in a considerable amount of time. Patients, or occasionally staff, colonized with highly antibiotic-resistant organisms, such as MRSA, may be important sources of cross-infection. Some of these highly-resistant organisms, e.g. MRSA and Gram-negative bacilli, may become untreatable in the future and every effort is required to eradicate them at an early stage. Some strains of enterococci are already resistant to all commonly used antibiotics.

Organization of infection control in the UK (Department of Health, 1995)

Infection Control Team (ICT)

The team consists of the Infection Control Doctor (ICD), Infection Control Nurse (ICN) and the hospital microbiologist if he/she is not the ICD. The team reports, through the ICD, either directly or via the committee, to the hospital Chief Executive or Senior Administrator (Figure 1.1). The team is responsible for all day-to-day aspects of infection control and for preparing and implementing the infection control programme and policies. It should also be associated with audits involving any aspects of infection control. The team liaises with all hospital departments and especially the Consultant in Communicable Disease Control (CCDC) or appropriate public health medical officer (see below). It is also responsible for surveillance of infection,

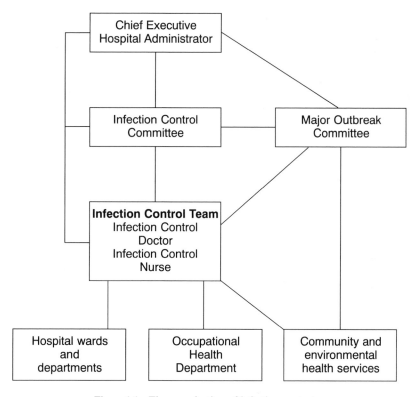

Figure 1.1   The organization of infection control

monitoring of hospital hygiene, investigating and advising on control of outbreaks and has an educational role for training all hospital staff in infection control. The team will usually meet daily or at least several times a week.

Infection Control Doctor

The ICD is usually a medically qualified microbiologist in the UK, but in some other countries may be an infectious diseases physician or epidemiologist and may be referred to as the Infection Control Officer (ICO) or hospital epidemiologist. In this book ICD will be used for the physician responsible for infection control. It is important that the ICD is a senior member of the hospital staff and is trained in infection control. The ICD will usually lead the infection control team and should have direct access to the hospital Chief Executive or Senior Administrator. He/she should liaise with the CCDC, especially in the investigation of outbreaks. The duties and responsibilities of the ICD are those of the team.

Infection Control Nurse

The ICN should be a registered nurse, preferably with experience in a relevant specialty, such as surgery, intensive care, paediatrics or infectious diseases. She/he is usually the only full-time member of the ICT and should attend an appropriate course, e.g. ENB 329 in the UK. Every major acute hospital should employ at least one ICN, and additional appointments should be made depending on the size of the hospital (e.g. two or three in the larger hospitals) and type of patient. The functions of the ICN are those of the team with special responsibilities for surveillance, implementation and audit of policies, staff education, nursing practices and day-to-day advice to staff. Liaison with all departments is an important aspect of the work and should include at least a daily visit to the laboratory. Since patients are being rapidly discharged from hospital to the community, consideration should be given to the appointment of ICNs with a specific role in the community.

Infection Control Link Nurses

Junior registered nurses working in a ward or unit may be given this part-time responsibility. They liaise with, and are responsible to, the ICN on infection control problems and provide information on infected patients and on problems with the implementation of policies. They are particularly useful in specialized units or units not on the main hospital site, but cannot replace trained ICNs. They should undergo a formal training programme, e.g. ENB N26 in the UK, and attend regular update workshops.

The medical staff also have a major role in the prevention of infection. It may be useful in some countries to appoint link clinical doctors as well as nurses, especially in high-risk units.

In some countries, another trained person, such as a laboratory scientist or pharmacist, is involved in infection control, often in addition to the the ICN and both scientists and nurses may be referred to as infection control practitioners (ICPs).

Consultant in Communicable Disease Control

This is a recent appointment in the UK. The CCDC is a physician with public health, microbiological and epidemiological training. He/she is responsible for the control of communicable diseases in the community and the hospital and is a member of the hospital Infection Control Committee. He/she also liaises with the ICT which retains responsibility for infection control in the hospital. The CCDC advises the local Health Authority on infection control aspects of contracts with individual hospitals and plays an important role in setting standards. In this book, CCDC will be used for the public health medical officer responsible for communicable diseases in the community and for control of major outbreaks of infectious diseases in both hospital and the community.

Infection Control Committee (ICC)

The ICC will usually be chaired by the ICD. The committee will consist of the Chief Executive or his representative, members of the ICT, the CCDC, a senior nurse and clinician and the Occupational Health Officer or nurse. Other staff, e.g. the Sterile Services Manager or the pharmacist, may be committee members or co-opted as necessary. The committee is responsible to the hospital Chief Executive or Senior Administrator for providing advice on major infection issues, especially if there are financial implications, and for ensuring that policies with infection control components (Table 1.3) exist in all appropriate departments of the hospital. It should also ensure that an up-to-date major outbreaks policy is available and that it is distributed to relevant staff. Major outbreaks are discussed in Chapter 4. A manual of policies will usually be produced by the ICT for committee approval. The committee should provide support to the ICT, but once policies are established need only meet once or twice a year or if required.

Table 1.3   Infection control administration

- *Organization*: Infection Control Team and Committee, Major Outbreaks Committee
- *Surveillance* and feedback of results
- *Formulation of policies*:
    Antibiotic, disinfectant, aseptic techniques, patient isolation
    Investigation and control of outbreaks, e.g. MRSA
    Decontamination of medical equipment
    Sharps and waste disposal, laundry, catering, infestation, health and safety
- *Implementation* of policies, audit
- *Staff immunization* (with Occupational Health Department)
- *Education and training of staff*

Other personnel and committees

Many hospitals have appointed other personnel with a specialized function which may be associated with infection control, e.g. risk management, audit, waste management, pest control, wound care and safety. Committees may also be formed to deal with these areas and could include reuse of disposables, waste management and safety.

A drugs and therapeutic committee is particularly important in defining antibiotic usage and agreeing on a policy. The committee should have the support of the medical staff, and a senior clinician should be a member; also the medical microbiologist should attend when antibiotics are being discussed.

The antibiotic policy should include the following:

- A list of restricted agents due to high cost or increasing antibiotic resistance. These should preferably not be purchased and, if prescribed, the pharmacist should inform the microbiologist or another member of the committee for discussion with the prescriber before the agent is issued.
- Junior medical staff should be trained in antibiotic usage and if possible provided with a handbook with the hospital recommendations for treatment of infections. The medical microbiologist should provide advice on treatment of individual patients and a member of the ICT should attend audit and clinical meetings where appropriate.
- Surgical prophylaxis should be restricted to one or two doses.
- The laboratory should restrict reporting of antibiotic sensitivity tests to recommended agents for the particular infection.
- Current antibiotic resistance patterns should be sent routinely to clinicians.
- In addition to control of antibiotics, the most important method of reducing the incidence of antibiotic resistance is the prevention of cross-infection. All staff need to be reminded of the necessity to wash their hands at the correct time.
- A quality control system of testing antibiotic sensitivities should be in place with reference laboratories to provide assistance and training where necessary.

The ICT should also liaise with the local Environmental Health Officers on catering and environmental hygiene and with the Health and Safety Executive on problems of staff safety.

Audit

The ICT should be involved in quality control in most of the departments in a hospital and should have an input into the methods of audit and their assessment. (Department of Health 1995) This should include laundry, catering, sterile supply services and waste management as well as clinical audit. The team should carry out its own audit procedures on infection control policies (see Table 1.3) in wards and other departments by means of questionnaires and observation. In addition, the team should audit its own standards of work, e.g. scope and quality of surveillance, quality and speed of advice, support to clinical and other staff and management of outbreaks.

Health services and infection control

The structure of the health services has changed in the UK in recent years. Local District Health Authorities and fund-holding general practitioners are responsible for purchasing care for patients in the hospitals and for some community services, but this system is likely to change again and all the general practitioners will probably have a greater role in purchasing care. The District Health Authority also has a responsibility for ensuring quality of care, which includes control of infection. The hospitals and community services are providers of care funded through annual contracts with the local Health Authorities or fund-holding general practitioners, although these funds are provided to the Health Authorities and general practitioners by government which provides central guidance. However, the requirement for annual contracts may cease and co-operation rather than competition between providers will be introduced. Hospitals controlled by a Chief Executive are usually trusts with responsiblility for their own affairs and for obtaining contracts for their services. The Chief Executive has the responsibility for ensuring the presence of an efficient infection control service and providing the ICT with adequate support, including additional funding for investigating and control of outbreaks when required. It is important that funding arrangements do not interfere with the vital role of microbiological specimens in the epidemiology of infectious disease. However, the Health Authority has overall responsibility for control of infectious diseases in hospitals and the community and operates through the CCDC and could provide additional funding for major outbreaks if necessary, particularly if more than one hospital and the community are affected.

Surveillance of hospital infection

To keep infection at a minimum level and to prevent and control outbreaks, some surveillance is necessary, even in hospitals in countries with few resources. This is not only to identify problems rapidly, but to ensure an adequate quality of care as far as prevention of infection is concerned (Emmerson and Ayliffe, 1996). Measurement of outcome, e.g. of patients in intensive care units or of patients who have undergone surgery, is important. It is possible, albeit crudely, to measure infection rates in an individual hospital, but comparisons of infection rates between hospitals are complex. Surveillance can be time consuming and is not always cost effective, particularly if the results are not used to improve infection control measures. The extent of surveillance depends on the resources available and it may be advisable to decide on priorities, e.g. high-risk units and antibiotic resistance, rather than covering a wider area superficially (Haley, 1995).

There are many definitions of surveillance, but most are similar. One of the more recent is 'the systematic, active, ongoing observation of the occurrence and distribution of disease in a population and response to the information collected' (modified from Hughes, 1987).

In practice, surveillance in a hospital comprises:

- the routine collection of data on hospital-acquired infection
- analysis of the data
- feedback of results to the ICC, clinicians and nursing staff.

The main purposes of surveillance are:

- to detect unusual levels or changes in the incidence of infection
- to identify hazardous or highly antibiotic-resistant organisms to enable early investigation and application of control measures
- to assess the efficacy of control measures.

Good surveillance can reduce infection rates. The Study on the Efficacy of Nosocomial Infection Control (SENIC), in the USA, carried out in 1975–80, showed that hospitals with active surveillance and control programmes could reduce the incidence of infection by 32%. This required an infection control physician and an infection control practitioner responsible for 250 beds (Haley et al., 1985). This reduction in infection associated with feedback to clinicians has been confirmed in other studies. The SENIC study was expensive and unlikely to be repeated, but was statistically sound. It remains uncertain why surveillance should reduce infection rates, but it seems likely that feedback of results was associated with improved techniques of clinical staff. The most cost-effective surveillance method for UK hospitals is unknown, but there are some useful comparisons of methods. Glenister et al. (1993) carried out a continuous prospective study of different selective methods of surveillance, i.e. laboratory-based ward, laboratory-based telephone, laboratory-based ward liaison, risk factor, temperature chart review and temperature chart and treatment chart review. These methods were compared with a reference method aimed at detecting all infections. The sensitivity of each method, i.e. the ability to identify patients with infections, and the specificity, i.e. the ability to identify patients without infection, were recorded as a percentage when compared with the reference method. The time taken to collect the data was also measured. The reference method consisted of the identification of all acquired infection.

Surveillance can be limited, e.g. based on daily examination of laboratory reports or routine visits to wards to question staff on the presence of infections, or quantitative, in which records are kept of all infections in a hospital, or targetted at special units only, or at certain procedures, e.g. surgical operations. These are either measurements of *incidence* which consist of the number of new cases in a defined population over a defined period, or *prevalence* which consists of the number of cases of acquired infection in a defined population during a specified period (period prevalence) or a specified point in time, e.g. one day (point prevalence). All patients in the hospital are visited on one occasion only and the presence of an infection recorded.

Prevalence surveys can be useful in that they can rapidly provide infection rates for the whole hospital and are less time consuming than continuous surveillance of all patients. However, the numbers of infections in individual surveys are small and no information is available on outbreaks occurring between surveys. Prevalence rates are usually about twice as high as incidence rates, since they incorporate the additional length of stay of infected patients. Prevalence rates in the hospital alone can be misleading if many of the patient population are undergoing day surgery or are discharged one or two days after operation or admission. Prevalence surveys can also be useful for identifying wards and hospitals with particular infection control problems and for assessing the impact of an infection control programme (French *et al.*, 1989). They are particularly useful for providing background information before setting up an infection control programme in a hospital with no previous infection control organization. Periodic prevalence surveys may be preferred to continuous surveillance of all patients if supported by some routine method of identifying outbreaks.

To obtain accurate surveillance results which can be compared with other hospitals for research purposes or in the same hospital at different times, the following are required:

- agreed definitions of infection (preferably nationally agreed)
- accurate denominator data
- correction of infection rates for risk factors, e.g. age, diabetes or other existing diseases, immunosuppression, type of operation, length of preoperative stay, length of time of catheterization (intravascular or urinary), and many others
- identification of hospital-acquired infections emerging after discharge from hospital.

The last item may be difficult to obtain accurately and the cost-effectiveness of collecting the information in the community requires further study. A national surveillance study (NINSS) is being carried out to provide information on infections in hospitals.

Risk factors can only be incorporated easily into surveillance results if all patient data are computerized, including the special factors related to infection. This would allow infections to be stratified according to risk or corrected by a computer model. Nevertheless, crude infection rates, e.g. surgical wounds, categorized by type of operation and whether clean, clean-contaminated or contaminated, can still be useful for infection control teams for internal audit, but not political use.

As indicated by the SENIC study, feedback of infections to the surgeons is necessary and should be supplied for clinical audit. It may be preferable that the surgeons should be responsible for their own infection records, with additional data provided by the ICT.

Some suggested surveillance methods which will depend on the availability of staff and resources are as follows:

1. *Hospitals with computerization of all patient data, including infection risk factors, and sufficient infection control and secretarial staff.* Continuous clinical and laboratory surveillance of all patients could be considered. This method is the 'gold standard' and will rarely be possible or necessary. It involves at least three visits a week to all wards by the ICN who reviews medical and nursing notes, including temperature charts, X-ray and laboratory reports, antibiotic administration and discussions with staff. This method is time consuming i.e. 18 h/week for 100 beds (Glenister *et al.*, 1993) and is usually not cost effective, since hospital infection will be infrequent in some wards. It may be preferable to target some wards, e.g. intensive care and surgical.

2. *Hospitals with a good laboratory and an ICT, but probably without full computerization of relevant patient risk factors.* Laboratory-based ward liaison may be appropriate. This consists of review of patients with positive laboratory reports by the ICN every day, and twice weekly visits to all wards to discuss all patients with the ward staff. This is time consuming (6.4 h/week for 100 beds) but is the most sensitive method (76%) after the reference method. It is probably the most cost-effective method, particularly if targeted at special wards. The success of the method depends on the ward staff taking appropriate samples and the accurate completion of laboratory report forms.

3. *Hospitals with good laboratory facilities, but with insufficient infection control staff to carry out overall continuous surveillance.* Laboratory-based ward surveillance is suggested. This consists of review of patients with positive laboratory reports and follow-up of infected patients. The method depends on the collection of samples as in method 2. However, additional infections can be detected by ICNs in discussion with ward staff.

4. *Hospitals with no full-time infection control staff and inadequate laboratory facilities.* Infections are recorded by a defined member of ward staff (e.g. a link nurse or doctor). Wards should regularly be visited by a person designated as responsible for infection control who will examine the records and check the results and take action if necessary.

5. *Other methods* can be used, e.g. infections in patients with known risk factors, patients on antibiotic therapy, patients with invasive devices or routine temperature chart review. These provide different but useful surveillance information and can be used alone or in combination with the methods described above.

Although infection control and patient information is often computerized, the data providing relevant information on risk factors and infections after discharge from hospital are rarely available for all patients, especially those without infection. Accurate infection rates are therefore not easily obtainable. However, useful surveillance data can be collected in most well-equipped hospitals.

Keeping accurate records is time consuming and only records on which action can be taken should be kept. ICNs should restrict their time spent on surveillance to not more than a couple of hours per day, otherwise other aspects of their work will suffer.

Most laboratories can record particularly hazardous or transmissible organisms and highly antibiotic-resistant strains, i.e. alert organisms (see Chapter 4). To improve the 'alert' organisms surveillance system, the following additions can be introduced:

- Examine laboratory records daily for wound infections, positive blood cultures, positive CSF cultures and infections in special units.
- ICN visits these wards to confirm they are clinical infections and hospital acquired. Question ward staff for the presence of other infections and, since laboratory specimens are not always sent, persuade them to send samples from any other infections (method 3, above).

- Ward staff should be trained to report 'alert' conditions, e.g. several cases of diarrhoea, to the ICT by telephone before the laboratory results are available.
- Visit special units daily or at least three times a week.

If sufficient ICNs are available, targeted surveillance using the laboratory-based/ward-liaison method may be carried out, e.g. surgical wounds, catheterized patients. Surveys of wards or procedures may be rotated as necessary.

Costs of hospital-acquired infection, cost effectiveness of infection control, legal implications and risk assessment

The main costs of hospital-acquired infection (HAI) can be calculated from the increase in length of stay and additional specific treatment, services or materials, e.g. antibiotics, disinfectants, protective clothing, dressings, infection control staff, but the true costs are difficult to quantify. The increased length of stay may not have such a great influence on actual costs in the UK National Health Service, but will influence the cost effectiveness of the service. If the patient pays for hospital stay, extra days in hospital could be costly. Indirect costs include microbiology and additional sterile supply services and isolation facilities. Disposal of clinical waste and environmental effects of incineration, especially of single-use plastics and the disposal of disinfectants, may all add ultimately to the costs of infection and its prevention. In addition, pain, inconvenience to patients and families, loss of earnings, loss of tax to the state and payment of sickness benefits can all be included as potential costs. In recent years, costs of claims for negligence have increased considerably and are diverting funds from necessary patient care. Mortality from hospital infection is low in most countries, but it is much more often a contributory factor to death from other causes.

A calculation in the UK based on an additional four days in hospital and an infection rate of 5% was assessed at £111 000 000 or 950 000 lost patient days in 1987. These estimates are very conservative and since then costs of hospital treatment have risen considerably, but with shorter hospital stay, costs of HAI may be transferred to the community. Little good evidence is available on the detailed costs of individual infections, and estimates of costs of infection from case control studies in various countries have varied, ranging from £250 to £2200 per patient (Department of Health, 1995). The extra days in hospital range from 2.4 for urinary tract infections to 17 for some orthopaedic operations. A study in the UK in 1988 on surgical wound infections showed an extra stay of 8.2 days and an additional cost per patient of £1041 (Coello *et al.*, 1993). Assuming that the study hospital was representative of other hospitals, the estimated costs of HAI occurring in similar patients throughout England amounted to £170 000 000.

Costs of HAI

Determining the cost of HAI is therefore fraught with difficulties. In the first instance the infections have to be identified, both those appearing in hospital and those continuing or appearing after discharge. HAI imposes additional direct costs, e.g. additional antibiotics; indirect costs (those related to, but not directly involved in, the episode, e.g. cleaning); and intangible costs such as those associated with pain and anxiety. These costs may fall on the health care sector (primary and secondary), on patients, on their family and friends, on social services, and on society as a whole, e.g. production losses.

Methods used to estimate costs have focused on the hospital sector. In particular they have attributed prolongation of stay wholly to HAI, and this is not necessarily the case. An episode of infection may occur, and be resolved, within the predicted period of treatment for that patient. Prolongation of stay may be for other clinical or social reasons. Charges, or prices, are not the same as costs, and this factor makes comparisons with other health care systems difficult (Plowman et al., 1997).

A study on the socio-economic burden of HAI has endeavoured to overcome the major methodological problems, and is awaiting publication. The majority of adult in-patients admitted to the non-specialist wards of a district general hospital over a 12-month period were recruited to the study – a total of nearly 4000. Cost profiles (including direct, indirect and intangible costs) incurred during the hospitalized phase and the first month post-discharge were collected for all study participants, whether or not they had a HAI. This method provided information on overall costs, on the unit costs and on the costs of infection, e.g. the cost of treatment of urinary tract infections. The results will allow infection control teams and managers to determine where the greatest morbidity and costs lie; to target their surveillance; and to use resources for prevention more effectively.

The study did not look at the cost of prevention of infection or at the effectiveness of prevention activities. Many of these are so deeply embedded in the hospital systems that they are difficult to unravel. For example, how much of the cost of providing handwashing facilities, hot water, soap and towels can be attributed to preventing infection, and how much to aesthetics? How much of the cost of providing hot water is for handwashing? In addition to the cost of prevention activities, the effectiveness of the interventions needs to be established. Daschner (1989) has examined the rationale and costs of some practices believed to prevent infection, and concluded that many are unproven or that cheaper alternatives exist. This aspect of infection control remains an area for extensive research.

Cost effectiveness of infection control

Hospital treatment is, amongst other things, an inefficient use of resources. It is in the interests of patients, clinicians, managers and funding bodies that it is reduced to a minimum (Dascher, 1989, Dascher and Dettenkofer, 1997). However, it must also be recognized that all infection cannot be prevented even if control methods are excellent. There is an irreducible minimum which it is impossible to avoid (Ayliffe, 1986) but is difficult to define. Many infections are endogenous in origin, i.e. acquired from the patient's own normal flora, and complete prevention of these is not possible. The SENIC study showed that an active surveillance and control programme with a physician and ICN could reduce infection rates by 32%, but even a reduction of 10% would more than cover the costs of an ICT (Wenzel, 1995). A study in Hong Kong showed a reduction in prevalence from 10.5% to 5.6% over 3 years following the introduction of an ICT and agreed control policies, with considerable overall annual savings ($6.9 million) (French *et al.* 1989). The number of outbreaks prevented is unknown and the possible savings made by an efficient infection control team could be considerable. Costs of outbreaks of methicillin-resistant *Staphylococcus aureus* are high and have been estimated as over £400 000 (Cox *et al.*, 1995).

ICTs can also save money by reducing rituals, e.g. discontinuing the routine use of disinfectants and encouraging better use of antibiotics.

There is obviously a need to identify those procedures most likely to be effective in prevention of infection and target them more precisely. A scientific, or at least a logical, explanation of how the proposed measures will reduce infection is required. For example, obtaining a reduction in the number of organisms in the environment may not be a sufficient reason to introduce a new measure if there is no evidence that the existing level of organisms has been responsible for infections. Whenever possible, resources should be allocated on a scientifically evaluated assessment and should be specifically targeted at the mode of spread (see Chapter 3). However, selection of priorities may be determined by other influences not necessarily within the control of the hospital administration, e.g. requirements of the Health and Safety Executive or local environmental health officers.

The introduction of clinical governance, evidence-based guidelines, standards, (Infection Control Working Party, 1993) and policies and legislation will help to prevent some of these problems. Locally based policies interpret national guidelines according to the local requirements.

Practice guidelines are 'systematically developed statements which assist practitioners and patients in making decisions about appropriate treatment for specific conditions' and are not legally enforceable. However, they are often used as a basis for prosecution by government agencies or in claims of negligence. Any deviation from national guidelines or standards requires some care, but it should be recognized that a consensus decision by a group of experts does not always indicate that it is the only or even the best solution. National guidelines should take into account differences between hospitals and where uncertainty exists should allow final decisions to be taken at a local level. Hospital policies may similarly be quoted in a court of law and it is important that these should be achievable in practice and implemented. Where possible they should have a scientific basis and be cost-effective. Guidelines should, if possible, indicate the strength of recommendations, e.g. randomized controlled trials, other robust experimental or observational studies or more limited evidence, but the advice relies on expert opinion and has the endorsement of respected authorities (NHS Executive, 1996). Other classifications are available, e.g. from the Centers for Disease Control in the USA (see Garner, 1996).

Legal implications

Costs of legal damages to hospital authorities can be very high. These can be lessened by good infection control practices. Patients now have a greater

expectation from treatment and are less likely to accept complications, such
as infection, as an acceptable risk. Some patients, particularly with certain
risk factors, are more likely to develop an infection, irrespective of apparently
adequate infection control measures. It is important that they are informed
of these potential risks before treatment. Clinicians and infection control
staff are required to maintain a duty of care, which means 'a duty to exercise
reasonable skill and care in the treatment of a patient or client'. The duty
of care applies also to the health and safety of staff, e.g. COSHH requirements
which include micro-organisms as well as use of disinfectants (see Chapter
8). Decisions made by a member of the infection control staff must therefore
be reasonable in the light of existing knowledge and commonly accepted
practice, even if the decision later turns out to be possibly incorrect; for
example, sending home a patient who is a salmonella carrier is accepted
practice, but this may be queried if other members of the family subsequently
acquire the infection. Many hospitals have a risk manager who can assist
the ICT. Negligence is usually associated with outdated knowledge or not
taking safety measures known to be necessary. It is important that hospital
policies are kept up to date, subjected to audit and followed by all staff. It
is accepted that there will often be disagreements on optimal procedures,
and the Bolam principle is accepted by legal authorities. This states: 'that a
practitioner is not guilty of negligence if he/she has acted in accordance with
a practice accepted as proper by a responsible body of medical men skilled
in that particular art. A doctor is not negligent if he is acting in accordance
with such a practice, merely because there is a body of opinion which takes
a contrary view.' Presumably this would apply to others who are expert in
their own right and make their own decisions, e.g. the ICN. This principle
would apply to infection control practices where there is often disagreement
between practitioners.

Risk assessment

Risk assessment has been an integral part of infection prevention and control
strategies since the concept of high-, medium- and low-risk equipment was
first introduced (see Chapter 9). Health care itself is a risk activity. Managing
risk has become a feature of health care activity, and the theme recurs
repeatedly throughout this text. The important feature is that risks should
be taken on the basis of sound information, not through ignorance or
passive acceptance, or some other driving force such as attempts to save
money. Daily risk management depends on harnessing the expertise of the
personnel employed by the organization. The ability to manage risks also
depends on the culture of the organization and, to some extent, on the
funding available.

   The principles of risk management are part of a cyclical process: identifying
the risk; analysing and evaluating its component parts; deciding whether to
accept the risk and its consequences, avoid the risk by transferring it, or
control the risk by managing it. It should be a multi-disciplinary process.
It is certainly fraught with tensions between competing interests, and subject
to the law of diminishing returns. One of the arts of infection control is
managing these tensions by assessing risks properly, knowing when to fight,

when to give in and when to transfer the risk; for example, when a real risk exists, which could have serious consequences for patients or staff or result in adverse publicity for the Trust, but the funding needed to manage the risk goes elsewhere. In that case, the risk may be transferred to the person or group that makes the funding decision. The corollary to that line of thinking is that the ICT must be very good at assessing risk.

References and further reading

Ayliffe, G.A.J. (1986) The irreducible minimum. *Infect. Cont.*, **7** (suppl.), 92–95.
Ayliffe, G.A.J., Lowbury, E.J.L., Geddes, A.M. and Williams, J.D. (1992) *Control of Hospital Infection: A Practical Handbook*, London, Chapman and Hall.
Coello, R., Glenister, H., Fereres, J. *et al.* (1993) The cost of infection in surgical patients: a case control study. *J. Hosp. Infect.*, **25**, 239–250.
Cox, R.A., Conquest, C., Mallaghan, C. and Marples, R.R. (1995) A major outbreak of methicillin-resistant *Staphylococcus aureus* caused by a new phage-type (EMRSA-16). *J. Hosp. Infect.*, **29**, 87–106.
Daschner, F.D. (1989) Cost effectiveness in hospital infection control – lessons for the 1990s. *J. Hosp. Infect.*, **13**, 325–336.
Daschner, F. and Dettenkoffer, M. (1997) Protecting the patient and the environment – new aspects and challenges in infection control. *J. Hosp. Infect.*, **36**, 7–15.
Department of Health (1995) *Hospital Infection Control: Guidance on the Control of Infection in Hospitals*, prepared by the Hospital Infection Working Group of the Department of Health and PHLS, London, Department of Health.
Emmerson, A.M., Ayliffe, G.A.J. (eds) (1996) *Surveillance of Nosocomial Infections*. Bailliere's Clin. Infect. Dis., 3, No. 2, London, Bailliere Tindall.
Emmerson, A.M., Enstone, J.E., Griffin, M. *et al.* (1996) Survey of infection in hospitals – overview of results. *J. Hosp. Infect.*, **321**, 175–190.
French, G.L., Wong, S.L., Cheng, A.F.B. and Donnan, S. (1989) Repeated prevalence surveys for monitoring effectiveness of hospital infection control. *Lancet* **2**, 1021–1023.
Garner, J.S. (1996) Guideline for isolation precautions in hospitals. *Infect. Cont. Hosp. Epidemiol.*, **17**, 53–80.
Glenister, H.M., Taylor, L.J., Bartlett, C.L.R. *et al.* (1993) An evaluation of surveillance methods for detecting infections in hospital inpatients. *J. Hosp. Infect.* **23**, 229–242.
Glynn, A., Ward, V., Wilson, J. *et al.* (1997) *Hospital-acquired Infection: Surveillance Policies and Practice*, a report of a study of the control of hospital-acquired infection in nineteen hospitals in England and Wales, London, Public Health Laboratory Service.
Haley, R.W. (1995) The scientific basis for using surveillance and risk factor data to reduce nosocomial infection rates *J. Hosp. Infect.*, **30** (suppl.), 3–14.
Haley, R.W., Culver, D.H., White, J.W. *et al.* (1985) The efficacy of infection surveillance and control programs in preventing nosocomial infections in US hospitals. *Am. J. Epidemiol.*, **121**, 182–205.
Hughes, J.M. (1987) Nosocomial infection surveillance in the United States: historical perspective. *Infect. Cont.*, **8**, 450–453.
Infection Control Working Party (1993) *Standards in Infection Control in Hospitals*, Southampton, Hobbs.
Mayon-White, R.J., Ducel, G.I., Keriselidze, T. and Tikhomirov, E. (1988) An international survey of the prevalence of hospital-acquired infection. *J. Hosp. Infect.*, **11** (suppl. A), 43–48.
Meers, P., McPherson, M. and Sedgwick, J. (1997) *Infection Control in Healthcare*, 2nd edn, Cheltenham, Stanley Thornes.
National Health Service Executive (1994) *Risk Management in the NHS*, London, Department of Health.

National Health Service Executive (1996) *Clinical Guidelines*, London, Department of Health.

Plowman, R.M., Graves, N. and Roberts, J.A. (1997) *Hospital-acquired Infection*, London, Office of Health Economics.

The Royal Society (1992) *Risk: Analysis, Perception and Management*, London, The Royal Society.

Wenzel, R.P. (1995) The economics of nosocomial infections. *J. Hosp. Infect.*, **31,** 79–87.

Wilson, J. (1995) *Infection Control in Clinical Practice*, London, Bailliere Tindall.

2

Micro-organisms and their properties

A micro-organism or microbe is a rather loose term for any plant or animal which cannot be seen without a microscope and does not form organized tissues as do higher plants and animals. They are usually single-celled but some organisms, particularly fungi, are more complex. Micro-organisms causing disease in man may be divided into four groups – bacteria, viruses, fungi and protozoa.

Bacteria

Bacteria are the main causes of hospital-acquired infection, although viruses may occasionally cause an epidemic, particularly in children's wards. Bacteria are single-celled and are measured in microns (μm, i.e. 0.001 mm). They are variable in size and shape (Figure 2.1); bacilli are rod-shaped 2–5 μm × 0.8 μm in diameter; cocci are 0.8–1 μm and may exist in pairs (diplococci), bunches (staphylococci) or chains (streptococci). Others may exist as curved rods (vibrios) or spirals (spirochaetes). Bacteria may have other structures, such as filaments or flagella, which enable them to move in fluids, or a mucoid layer or capsule which protects some organisms, e.g. *Streptococcus pneumoniae* and *Klebsiella pneumoniae*, from the body defence mechanisms. Thick-walled structures (spores) may increase the resistance of certain bacteria, e.g. *Clostridium tetani, Cl. perfringens* and *Bacillus subtilis*, to moderate degrees of heat or to chemical disinfectants.

Bacteria usually multiply by binary fission, i.e. each organism increases in size, and then divides into two daughter cells. Other mechanisms of transferring genetic material may occur. In conjugation, two cells come together and genetic material (extrachromosomal) in a plasmid passes from one to another along a hollow tube or pilus. Conjugation is particularly important as resistance to antibiotics may be transferred by this method. Other methods of transfer of genetic material may take place, e.g. by a bacteriophage (transduction) or in deoxyribonucleic acid (DNA) from disrupted cells (transformation). Genetic material may also be transferred by transposons (jumping genes) from plasmids to chromosomes or vice versa, or to plasmids and chromosomes of other species.

Bacteria are found everywhere – in the air, in soil and water – and few are pathogenic (capable of producing disease in man). They are present in

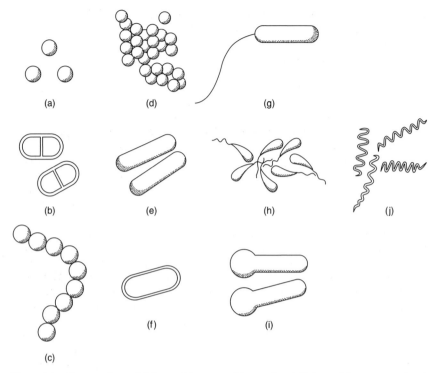

Figure 2.1   Common bacterial forms: (a) coccus; (b) capsulated diplococci (pneumococci); (c) cocci in chains (streptococci); (d) cocci in clusters (staphylococci); (e) bacillus; (f) capsulated bacilli (e.g. *Klebsiella* spp.); (g) bacillus with polar flagellum (e.g. *Pseudomonas* spp.); (h) curved bacilli (e.g. *Vibrio* spp.); (i) spore-bearing bacillus (e.g. *Clostridium* spp.); (j) spiral (spirochaetes)

the normal flora of the skin, in the mouth, vagina and the gastrointestinal tract. Organisms found on the skin are mainly *Staphylococcus epidermidis*, micrococci and diphtheroids (aerobic and anaerobic). *Streptococcus viridans, Moraxella catarrhalis* and anaerobic bacilli are found normally in the mouth and throat. *Escherichia coli, Proteus mirabilis, Klebsiella aerogenes, Enterobacter* spp., enterococci and anaerobic Gram-negative bacilli (*Bacteroides*) are found in the lower intestinal tract. The organisms of the normal flora do not usually cause disease in the sites where they normally exist and tend to protect the host from other organisms. However, they may cause infection in other sites, e.g. *E. coli* in the urinary tract, *Strep. viridans* or *Staph. epidermidis* in subacute endocarditis, and *Bacteroides* spp. may cause wound infection after operations on the colon or rectum.

Bacteria can be initially classified by their staining reaction. The Gram stain is the most useful. Gram-positive organisms stain a purplish-blue and include streptococci, staphylococci, aerobic and anaerobic sporing bacilli, e.g. *Bacillus subtilis, Clostridium perfringens* and *Cl. tetani*. Gram-negative organisms stain red and include some cocci, *Neisseria gonorrhoeae, N. meningitidis*, most of the aerobic bacilli, e.g. *E. coli, Klebsiella*, and anaerobic non-sporing bacilli. Some organisms, such as *Mycobacterium tuberculosis*, may be identified by a special stain. Mycobacteria are acid-fast and show as red bacilli on a blue or green background in a Ziehl–Neelsen stain. *Corynebacterium diphtheriae* show granules on staining by Albert's or Neisser's stain.

Direct staining of specimens is of limited value, but may sometimes assist in immediate diagnosis and treatment. Staphylococci or pneumococci may be recognized in purulent sputum and this may assist in the rapid diagnosis of pneumonia. A direct film may be useful in diagnosing a urinary tract infection but is of little value for making decisions on the choice of an antibiotic. Some bacteria may be directly identified by immunological tests, e.g. using monoclonal antibodies.

The sample, e.g. swab, pus, urine, etc., is cultured on a plate (petri dish) containing artificial media. The medium is basically a nutrient broth solidified if necessary by a gelatin-like substance – agar. The nutrient broth provides protein, carbohydrate, essential salts and other factors at a pH suitable for bacterial growth. Most bacteria isolated from human beings or animals either require blood for their growth, or show an improved growth on blood-containing media. A blood-agar plate, nutrient broth with agar and horse-blood, is commonly used and haemolysis of the blood can help in recognition of the organisms. When the plate is incubated at 37°C for 18–24 h, bacteria grow as colonies, each containing millions of organisms. Other types of media are used; MacConkey medium (bile-salt lactose agar) is useful for intestinal organisms. Other media are selective for pathogens, e.g. deoxycholate – citrate agar, for isolation of salmonellae or shigellae from faeces. In recent years anaerobes have increased in importance and are recognized by growth on plates incubated in the absence of oxygen.

Further tests may be necessary to identify organisms and include biochemical, e.g. fermentation of sugars, and serological to identify specific strains of salmonella or shigella. Antibiotic sensitivity tests may sometimes assist in identification.

The common organisms causing hospital infection and their properties are shown in Table 2.1.

The growth of bacteria in solutions is relevant to many problems in hospital infection. Typically in nutrient broth, there is a latent period lasting for 2–4 h in which no growth occurs, followed by a logarithmic phase of rapid growth, a stationary phase, and later a phase of decline when the organisms begin to die (Figure 2.2).

A similar growth pattern may be seen in urine and demonstrates the reason for examining urines within 2–3 h before growth occurs. Refrigeration at 4°C will prevent the organism from growing. Similar principles apply to the growth of bacteria in food which should be stored at temperatures below 5°C or above 63°C. Most bacteria fail to grow above 50°C except for some thermophilic strains, e.g. *Bacillus stearothermophilus*, which are non-pathogenic. The growth cycle described occurs in optimal conditions of temperature and nutrients and for most human pathogens this is between 35°C and 38°C. However, growth may be observed at lower temperatures (e.g. 20–25°C) but may take several days to reach the stationary phase. Some organisms, particularly *Klebsiella* and *Enterobacter* spp., are able to grow in the environment and may reach large numbers in 24 h with minimal nutrients. *Pseudomonas aeruginosa* can also grow to large numbers at room temperature in 24–48 h water. This explains the heavy growth of this

Table 2.1   Organisms and infections

Organisms	Infection	Main characteristics
Gram-positive		
Staphylococcus aureus	Boils, wounds, osteomyelitis, food poisoning	Coagulase-positive, usually resistant to benzylpenicillin
Staphylococcus epidermidis	Intravenous sites, endocarditis, wounds	Coagulase-negative
Streptococcus pyogenes (Group A)	Tonsillitis, scarlet fever, burns and puerperal infection	Clear beta-haemolysis on blood agar, sensitive to benzylpenicillin
Enterococcus	Urinary tract, subacute endocarditis	Usually sensitive to ampicillin (not benzylpenicillin), some strains are highly resistant to antibiotics
Clostridium perfringens	Gas gangrene, food poisoning	Anaerobic sporing bacillus, sensitive to benzylpenicillin
Clostridium tetani	Tetanus	Anaerobic, drum-stick spores, usually sensitive to benzylpenicillin
Clostridium difficile	Pseudomembramous colitis, antibiotic-associated diarrhoea	Sensitive to vancomycin and metronidazole
Gram-negative		
Escherichia coli	Urinary tract, wounds, pelvic sepsis	LF, usually sensitive to commonly used antibiotics
Klebsiella spp.	Urinary tract, wounds respiratory tract	LF. ampicillin-resistant
Proteus mirabillis	Urinary tract, wounds	NLF, typical smell, resistant to tetracycline and nitrofurantoin
Pseudomonas aeruginosa	Wounds, burns, urinary tract, chest	NLF, typical smell, green pigment
Enterobacter spp.	Urinary tract and wounds	NLF, resistant to cephalosporins
Salmonella spp.	Enteric fever, food poisoning	NLF, motile
Shigella spp.	Dysentery	NLF, non-motile
Campylobacter spp.	Diarrhoea	NLF
Acinetobacter spp.	Urinary tract, wounds respiratory tract,	NLF, often resistant to usual antibiotics
Serratia marcescens	Urinary tract, wounds, respiratory tract	NLF, often red colonies, usually resistant to cephalosporins
Legionella pneumophila	Respiratory tract	Requires special media
Bacteroides spp.	Wounds, pelvic sepsis, lung abscess	Anaerobic, non-sporing

LF, lactose fermenter; NLF, non-lactose fermenter.

organism obtained in washing bowls, shaving brushes, humidifiers, mops or endoscopes, which have not been adequately disinfected or dried. Other pseudomonads are able to grow in weak disinfectant solutions and have been reported in solutions of quaternary ammonium compounds, chlorhexidine, hexachlorophane, and occasionally in phenolics.

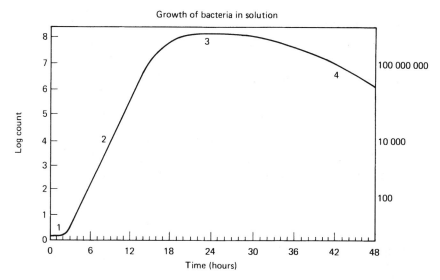

Figure 2.2   Growth of bacteria in a solution: 1, lag phase; 2, logarithmic growth phase; 3, stationary phase; 4, decline phase

Gram-negative bacilli can often adapt themselves to grow in concentrations of disinfectant which would normally kill them in laboratory tests. This is likely if solutions are topped-up when the container is empty instead of cleaning it and completely replacing with a new solution. This tends to occur with handwashing soaps or disinfectant solutions unless a suitable preservative is added. Contamination of tanks of disinfectant used for urine bottles has been reported because of topping-up rather than replacing the disinfectant solution. Dilute solutions of disinfectants are also often unstable.

Bacteria vary in their ability to grow in fluids. Staphylococci fail to grow in dextrose–saline at room temperature, whereas *Klebsiella* and *Serratia* spp. grow well. The risks of infection from intravenous fluids are much greater with these Gram-negative bacilli than with most other potential pathogens such as staphylococci, *E. coli*, etc. which require a higher temperature and additional nutrients to grow properly. Airborne organisms from the skin, e.g. coagulase-negative staphylococci, are only likely to get into intravenous fluids in small numbers when a container is opened for the addition of other fluids and are unlikely to grow. Greater care is necessary with intravenous alimentation therapy as sufficient nutrient is available for other organisms, such as *Candida*, to grow; additions to these fluids should be made in a laminar flow cabinet in the pharmacy, unless the fluid is used within a few hours.

Biofilms

Many hospital-acquired infections are associated with invasive devices. Tubing or catheters inserted into the intravascular system, into body cavities, e.g. in continuous ambulatory peritoneal dialysis (CAPD), central nervous system (CNS) shunts, urinary catheters and endotracheal tubes, may become colonized with bacteria and may be associated with clinical infection. Bacteria initially adhere to the surface of the device and form microcolonies which generate a matrix of slime (exopolysaccharide). This is termed a biofilm and its formation depends on a number of factors, e.g. the type and properties of the organism, the type of surface, the presence of nutrients and, where relevant, the velocity of flow of fluids over the surface. Bacteria will attach to and colonize any suitable surface with which they have contact and this includes mucous membranes as well as inanimate surfaces (Costerton *et al.*, 1995). The bacteria are protected by the biofilm from chemotherapeutic agents and host defences. The longer the devices remain in situ, the greater is the likelihood of biofilm formation and subsequent infection. Removal of the device as soon as possible is the most effective preventive measure.

Coagulase-negative staphylococci and Gram-negative bacilli are commonly associated with biofilm formation on medical devices. Coagulase-negative staphylococci are normal inhabitants of the skin and spread along the outer surface and sometimes along the lumen of intravenous catheters, forming a biofilm of slime often in association with fibrin and other proteins which are coating the catheter. Although colonization of the catheter is not in itself harmful, local infection can occur and small pieces of biofilm released into the bloodstream may be responsible for bacteraemia and less frequently septicaemia or endocarditis. Biofilms containing coagulase-negative staphylococci and sometimes *Staph. aureus* may also form on the surface of cardiac and artifical joint implants, causing infections which are difficult to treat and often requiring removal of the device.

Colonization with Gram-negative bacilli is particularly likely if the surface is in contact with non-sterile fluid. In tubing or pipes, the flow of the fluid tends to be less at the periphery. Nutrients and organisms will therefore accumulate at the surface of the tube and form a biofilm. As the biofilm increases in depth, free organisms will be released into the surrounding fluid. As the flow increases, the biofilm may be reduced due to the removal of organisms and slime by flushing. However, sampling of water supplies or washings from endoscopes may not provide accurate information on numbers of organisms if they are mainly present in biofilms and are not removed by rinsing alone.

Biofilms of Gram-negative bacilli form on the outer and inner surfaces of indwelling urinary catheters and spread to the bladder mucosa. Bacteriuria, and occasionally clinical infection, is almost inevitable with long-term catheterization. The biofilm can also bind crystals, causing obstruction of the catheter. Treatment with antibiotics or other chemotherapeutic agents is usually unsuccessful while the catheter remains in situ.

Endotracheal tubes can become colonized with antibiotic-resistant Gram-negative bacilli from the oropharynx and form a biofilm. As with urinary catheters, colonization alone does not require treatment, but infection can develop particularly in susceptible patients, e.g. comatosed patients or those on prolonged intubation, and is difficult to treat successfully.

Mycobacterium spp. (other than *M. tuberculosis)* and Gram-negative bacilli, especially *Legionella* and *Pseudomonas* spp., are commonly isolated from natural water supplies. These organisms may be present in large numbers in biofilms in association with many other organisms (e.g. amoebae, other protozoa and algae) in pipes and shower heads, particularly if the

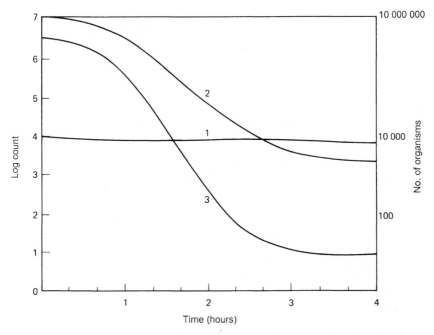

Figure 2.3 Survival of organisms on drying. Suspensions of organisms allowed to dry at room temperature over 4 h. 1, Spores survive well; 2, *Staph. aureus* shows moderate survival; 3, *Ps. aeruginosa* (and other Gram-negative bacilli) rapidly die on drying

water flow is slow or static as in deadlegs, in cooling towers and in poorly designed calorifiers. Legionella present in biofilms of water supplies may be further protected by their ingestion in amoebae. Apart from legionella, most of the organisms are not usually of medical significance, other than in endoscopes or washing machines. Biofilms containing mycobacteria or pseudomonads may be found in the water supply, tubing and rinse-water tank of endoscope washing machines and may recontaminate a bronchoscope after disinfection. The organisms can be transferred from a contaminated bronchoscope to bronchial washings and may be responsible for a pseudodiagnosis of infection. This is a particular hazard if acid-fast bacilli are found in the washings. *Ps. aeruginosa* from a contaminated endoscope has also caused infection in susceptible patients, e.g. leukaemics, or following an ERCP.

Effect of drying on survival

Although some Gram-negative bacilli can grow in fluids with minimal nutrients at room temperature, they are very susceptible to drying. *E. coli, Pseudomonas, Klebsiella*, and some other organisms, such as *Candida*, die rapidly on drying (Figure 2.3), but staphylococci show greater survival (Pettit and Lowbury, 1968). The implications are that Gram-negative bacilli rarely spread in the air, unless in an aerosol, whereas the airborne route is a more likely mode of spread for staphylococci. Nevertheless, staphylococci die on dry surfaces over several days and even after overnight the numbers are considerably reduced (Ayliffe *et al.*, 1967). The risks of transfer from the inanimate environment are small, even though some cells survive for months. Spore-bearing bacilli also survive well in the dry environment but are usually non-pathogenic, e.g. *B. subtilis.* Clostridia are commonly isolated in the dry environment of the hospital, usually in small numbers, but rarely cause a problem. However, *Cl. difficile* may be widely distributed in the inanimate environment. Beta-haemolytic streptococci survive poorly on drying, but large numbers have been found on blankets and in dust during outbreaks of infection. However, in recent years environmental contamination with β haemolytic streptococci has not been apparent in our experience.

A small number of Gram-negative bacilli will survive drying if the initial number of organisms is large, and they are protected by organic matter. This explains why *Ps. aeruginosa* can often be isolated from floors in burns units and possibly why airborne spread of enteropathogenic *E. coli* or *Salmonella* has occasionally been reported. Some Gram-negative bacilli, e.g. epidemic strains of *Klebsiella* and *Acinetobacter* spp. survive drying better than others. This may have epidemiological significance by improving their chance of spread on the hands. From the evidence available, thorough washing and drying is the best method of reducing any small risks of spread from the dry environment. Storing nail-brushes and thermometers in fluids has always been a potential hazard, particularly if fresh solutions are not made up daily. Common source outbreaks of *Pseudomonas* infection are now much less common since equipment is more often stored in a dry state. The relevance of these properties to the spread of infection will be considered in a later chapter.

Viruses

Viruses are small infective particles 20–200 nm in size (1000 nm = 1 μm, which is the size of a staphylococcal cell) and can only grow in living cells. Viral disease can be diagnosed by growing viruses in tissue cultures or by serological tests. Monoclonal antibodies are increasingly being used for rapid diagnosis of viral infections, e.g. by immunofluorescence. The survival of viruses in the environment is generally poor, and close contact is usually necessary for transmission. However, if large numbers are dispersed into the environment some will survive for relatively long periods. Hepatitis B virus (HBV) will survive for up to 7 days or longer. Human immunodeficiency virus (HIV), a retrovirus causing AIDS, will similarly survive for several days in the environment. Some viruses have a lipid capsule (enveloped viruses), e.g. herpes simplex and HIV, and are very susceptible to drying and disinfectants. Non-enveloped viruses, e.g. enteroviruses, survive better in the environment and are more resistant to disinfectants. Viruses are not a major cause of endemic infection in hospital but outbreaks of childhood viral infections (e.g. respiratory syncytial virus) can cause problems in paediatric wards. Some viruses, such as herpes simplex or zoster and cytomegalovirus, are particularly hazardous in immunosuppressed patients.

Prions

These are often termed 'slow viruses', but appear to be self-replicating proteins without detectable RNA or DNA. They have not been grown in tissue culture and are resistant to routine autoclaving and dry heat sterilization, ethylene oxide, glutaraldehyde and most other disinfectants, except high concentrations of chlorine-releasing agents and sodium hydroxide. They survive in formalin-fixed tissues (see p. 166).

Fungi

These are more complex structures than bacteria and may grow as filaments (mycelia) and produce reproductive spores. They can be grown on inanimate culture media, such as Sabouraud's agar. They are identified by their microscopic appearance, colonial morphology and sometimes by biochemical and serological tests. *Candida albicans* is the commonest fungus causing infection in hospital and may spread in neonatal units. It usually infects debilitated patients. Other fungi may cause infection in hospital but mostly in immunosuppressed patients. *Aspergillus fumigatus* is an example. Other fungi are rare, e.g. *Cryptococcus neoformans* may be found in the compromised host. It is found in bird droppings but whether this is a source of infection in hospital is uncertain. Aspergilli are common airborne contaminants and possibly isolating the compromised patient in a room with filtered air may reduce the likelihood of infection.

Protozoa

Protozoa are single-celled members of the animal kingdom and are rarely a cause of hospital infection. It is possible that malaria could be transferred in transfused blood but is very rare in Northern Europe and the USA. *Entamoeba histolytica*, a causative organism of dysentery, is also not readily directly transferred from person to person in hospital. Other protozoa tend to be found mainly in the compromised host, but the organisms are already present in the host and are reactivated due to immunological incompetence. *Pneumocystis carinii, Toxoplasma gondii, Giardia lamblia* and cryptosporidia are examples of protozoa causing infection in these patients. Cryptosporidia and *Giardia* may be responsible for water-borne infections.

Laboratory testing of microbiology specimens

Laboratory tests are time consuming and expensive and unnecessary tests should be avoided. Common reasons for wastage of resources are: unsuitable or unnecessary specimens, inadequate information on laboratory request forms, reports of little or doubtful value to the clinician. Identification and investigation of outbreaks depend on reliable laboratory tests (McGowan and Metchcock, 1996).

Collection of specimens

Pus should be sent to the laboratory whenever available; swabs taken from the pus are of less value. Many organisms, e.g. β-haemolytic streptococci, die rapidly on dry swabs. Pus or swabs in transport media should be sent to the laboratory as soon as possible if anaerobic culture is required.

'Sputum' consisting of saliva only is useless and reports are misleading. Urine is a good culture medium and should be sent to the laboratory or refrigerated within 2 h of collection or a preservative is added. Dip-slides may be preferable if rapid delivery to the laboratory or refrigeration is not possible. CSF and other fluids should be delivered as soon as possible to the laboratory as cells tend to disintegrate rapidly and delicate pathogens, e.g. *N. meningitidis*, may die. Samples of faeces are preferable to rectal swabs, but if swabs are taken they should show the presence of faeces; anal swabs (instead of rectal) are usually useless and may be misleading.

Containers for specimens should be filled aseptically to avoid contamination from organisms on the outside of the container, also to prevent contamination of the outside from organisms in the specimen. False outbreaks of infection have occurred due to collection of samples from several patients in the same unsterile container, e.g. urine in a bowl or jug, before transfer to the sterile laboratory container.

Viruses survive poorly on dry swabs and samples (swabs and washings) should be collected in special transport media and taken to the laboratory as soon as possible. If in doubt consult the laboratory; often laboratory personnel will prefer to collect their own specimens. Many virus infections can only be diagnosed serologically; blood from acute and convalescent stages of disease is required to demonstrate at least a four-fold rise in antibody titre.

It is most important that samples are taken before treatment is started. If septicaemia is suspected, two or more blood cultures should be taken at short intervals between them; treatment need not be delayed beyond 30 min.

Samples should also be correctly taken. Nose swabs should be moistened in sterile saline and rubbed several times firmly around each of the anterior nares. Throat swabs should be taken from the inflamed area, preferably obtaining some exudate. Contamination with saliva should be avoided. Careful cleaning of the vulva is necessary when collecting a mid-stream specimen of urine from a female. In general, superficial contamination should be avoided when collecting samples from infected lesions. Occasionally invasive techniques are necessary to obtain adequate or non-contaminated specimens, e.g. transtracheal aspiration, suprapubic puncture, aspiration of abscess. Bacterial counts on respiratory secretions are preferred to qualitative reports in the diagnosis of hospital-acquired pneumonia, e.g. on bronchial washings. Protective sampling devices are commonly used.

Specimens should only be sent if the results are likely to provide or confirm a diagnosis or exclude a likely diagnosis. Routine screening is rarely a cost-effective exercise and if undertaken should only be carried out in consultation with the microbiologist. All routine screening programmes should be checked at intervals of not more than 3 months. This will often show that either sufficient evidence is already available or that positive tests are so rare that continuation cannot be justified on cost alone or that treatment can be decided by alternative means.

When doubt exists the laboratory should always be consulted so that the most suitable specimen and method of collection can be agreed, and that the needs of the patient and priorities of the laboratory can be taken into consideration. All specimens are put through a routine procedure which will not always provide the answer to a specific problem. The microbiologist should be consulted about any problem patient. If the patient is responsible for costs of specimens, appropriate alternative arrangements should be made for epidemiological samples.

Inadequate information on request forms

Forms should be carefully designed so that the required information is likely to be provided by the clinician. The following information is necessary:

1. Age of patient: host susceptibility and diseases vary with age.
2. Name and number: the patient's hospital number should always be included. Names are often the same and mistakes can occur.
3. Ward: this is needed so that infection control staff can detect outbreaks, as well as ensuring the report is returned without delay.
4. Relevant history: this is most important as tests may be decided on this. A swab from a patient with puerperal sepsis is treated differently from one with a vaginal discharge. Writing 'wound swab' may waste time if it is really from a pressure sore. The cause of infection might be anaerobic and a suitable culture might not be made.
5. Site of infection: different areas of the body tend to have their own flora and the same organisms elsewhere may have a pathogenic role. *Staph. aureus* may be a normal inhabitant of the nose, but not in an infected finger.
6. Antibiotic therapy: failure to include this information often leads to a misleading report. The antibiotic may inhibit growth of the causative organism or select resistant strains which colonize the site, e.g. ampicillin-resistant klebsiellas are common in sputa of patients treated with ampicillin but are not necessarily a cause of clinical lung disease.
7. Date and time of collection: different organisms survive for varying periods and some grow well at room temperature. Sputa left overnight may show a heavy growth of *Candida* which is not significant. Even if a swab is placed in transport medium some Gram-negative bacilli may grow over several days.

Environmental sampling

Bacteria are normally present, often in large numbers, in an occupied environment. The types and numbers of organisms depend on the number of people occupying the area and their activity, the proportion of each sex present, the flow of air and the humidity. Bacterial counts of the air can change rapidly depending on circumstances. In general, the patient is much more likely to contaminate the environment than to be infected from it. For these reasons environmental sampling is of limited value, since numbers of bacteria are not necessarily related to hazards of infection.

Routine sampling of air and surfaces in operating theatres, wards, catering areas, sterile services departments and pharmacies is of little value. If a sampling programme is agreed it should be justified and have a specific objective; possible reasons are:

- to identify routes of spread of infection
- to identify staphylococcal dispersers
- to evaluate cleaning or disinfection techniques
- for research or teaching purposes.

When such procedures are required, the microbiologist should be consulted as interpretation requires experience in this field.

Sampling may be requested on commissioning of operating theatres (see Chapter 16).

Sampling techniques

Swabbing of surfaces, unless taken from a defined area using a standard technique, will indicate only the presence or absence of a limited range of organisms. Growth of *Cl. perfringens* from a broth culture of a swab taken from the floor of an operating theatre is no reason for closing the theatre suite.

Contact plates give a semi-quantitative result and are useful for comparing surfaces and also indicate the distribution of organisms on the surface. The technique is useful for detecting the presence of a staphylococcal disperser and large numbers of samples can be rapidly taken from surfaces. Separate plates are, of course, necessary for aerobic and anaerobic organisms. Contact plates are unsuitable for counting very large numbers of organisms and may show a semi-confluent or confluent growth. Washings from a defined area of a surface remove more organisms, and also tend to break up clumps, giving much higher counts than contact plates. More accurate counts are obtained, especially with large numbers of organisms, but give no indication of spatial arrangement.

Air samples are usually measured with a slit sampler or by exposing settle plates. The slit sampler demonstrates the number of colony-forming units in the air, but many may be small particles which would not fall into a wound. Sizes of bacteria-carrying particles can be measured with an Anderson or a Cascade sampler. Several portable samplers are now available, but volumes of air sampled may be too low for some investigations.

Settle plates measure the bacteria-carrying particles falling onto the plate over a defined period but not the total numbers in the air. However, this is a simple technique and is useful for identifying staphylococcal dispersers in a ward or theatre.

Fluids should be sampled with a pipette and total organisms counted. It is important that whenever the environment is sampled, the technique used should be quantitative or semi-quantitative if any useful conclusions are to be made from the observations.

Typing of bacteria

Most infections acquired in hospital are caused by organisms which are part of the normal flora, e.g. *Staph. aureus* or *E. coli*, or are commonly found in the environment, e.g. *Kl. aerogenes* or *Ps. aeruginosa*.

Ps. aeruginosa can be found in 25% or more of hospital sinks but these strains are usually of different types from those causing infections (Lowbury *et al.*, 1970). *Staph. aureus* is present in the noses of 20% of healthy people and typing studies have shown that strains isolated from ward nurses are not common causes of wound infections. The identification of the species in these instances is rarely of value. It therefore may be necessary to use additional methods, e.g. typing, to establish whether strains have originated from a single source or are epidemiologically related. On the other hand, the isolation of an unusual organism, such as *S. typhi*, from two or more patients in a ward is highly suggestive of cross-infection without the necessity of additional typing methods.

In typing systems, specific markers of organisms are used which are characteristic of a single strain or clone (indicating that the organisms are derived from the same precursor cell), and which differ from other strains. The methods commonly used are biotyping, antibiograms, resistotyping, phage, bacteriocin and serological typing, and more recently molecular typing (Struelens, 1996). The usefulness of a typing system depends on its reproducibility, discriminating ability, stability and the percentage of typable strains. For instance, a system in which only 50% of strains are typable (poor typability), or 60% are of the same type (poor discrimination) or the same result is not obtained on each occasion in the same or indifferent laboratories (poor reproducibility), is not likely to be a very useful system.

Biotyping

This method is an extension of the biochemical techniques commonly used for identification of species, i.e. enzyme production, fermentation of sugars, as already described. It is of limited value in the subdivision of species, but may be useful for characterizing organisms such as *Acinetobacter* spp., *E. coli* or coagulase-negative staphylococci where other typing methods are not available in a routine laboratory. A wide range of tests is usually necessary, e.g. over 20, making this a rather expensive method. Occasionally a strain may have an unusual property, such as indole-positive *Klebsiella*, spp. which enables it to be sufficiently well characterized for epidemiological purposes in an outbreak in one ward, but not as a general typing method. Commercial systems, such as the API, are now commonly used in laboratories.

Diene's test
This is a useful test for differentiating strains of *Proteus mirabilis*. A line of inhibition is seen between spreading haloes of different strains of *P. mirabilis* on an agar plate. No zone of inhibition is seen when the spreading halves are from the same strain.

Antibiograms and resistograms

Antibiograms are of limited use, as many strains show similar patterns. Many staphylococcal wound infections are caused by strains resistant to penicillin only and *Kl. aerogenes* tends to be resistant to the common antibiotics, and differences between strains are often not sufficient to characterize individual strains. However, some strains of *Staph. aureus* or Gram-negative bacilli are resistant to four or five antibiotics and this may be sufficient to identify a strain in a ward. It is likely, although not certain, that strains of *Staph. aureus* resistant to methicillin, gentamicin, erythromycin and tetracycline isolated from several patients in a ward are the same strain. Occasionally resistance to a single antibiotic may be equally useful. Gentamicin resistance in *Ps. aeruginosa* may be sufficient evidence to suggest a single strain is spreading in a unit, but is not entirely reliable. Antibiotic resistance is usually controlled by a plasmid, which can be transferred between genera as well as species, and plasmids can be lost so that antibiograms must be used with caution in identifying single strains. Nevertheless, determining the antibiotic resistance pattern is one of the most useful typing methods in routine laboratories.

Resistograms are similar to antibiograms except sensitivity is measured to a range of chemicals (Phelps *et al.*, 1986). Although this method is useful for typing organisms, such as *E. coli, Proteus* or *Candida*, for which other methods are not readily available, it is difficult to control. Most laboratories could use this method, but the requirement is so rare that it is not usually worth setting it up as a routine procedure.

Serological typing

In this method a range of specific antisera is used to detect surface antigens characteristic of a particular species, or to subdivide a single species for epidemiological purposes.

It is commonly used for routinely identifying species, particularly *Salmonella* and *Shigella*. Since more than one strain, e.g. *Salmonella typhimurium*, is unlikely to be in a ward at the same time, identification other than of the species is usually sufficient. Additional typing may be necessary in the community where it may be useful to determine the source of a strain of *Salmonella*, e.g. in an outbreak of food poisoning, a particular food type, animal or a certain farm is suspect. However, serological typing of commonly isolated strains such as *Klebsiella* and *Ps. aeruginosa* can be of considerable value in investigating outbreaks of hospital infection. Serological types are usually stable, but sometimes serotyping must be combined with other methods, such as phage or bacteriocin, as some serotypes are particularly common.

Haemolytic streptococci can be usefully subdivided into groups, i.e. Lancefield A, B, C, D, and these can be further subdivided into Griffiths types.

Phage typing

Phages are small viruses which grow in bacterial cells and usually destroy them. A typical phage is shown in Figure 2.4. It consists of a head containing deoxyribonucleic acid (DNA) and a tail. The hollow tail attaches itself to

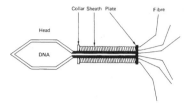

Figure 2.4   Diagram of phage

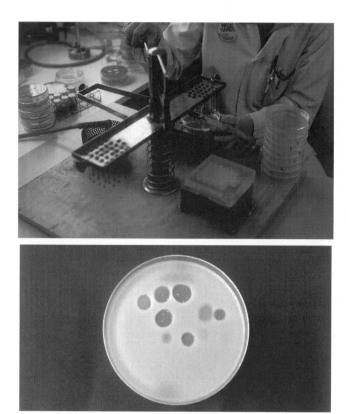

Figure 2.5   (a) Phage typing. (b) Plate showing pattern of lysis

the bacterial wall and DNA passes along it into the bacterial cells. The phage DNA takes over the DNA-producing mechanism of the bacterial cell and makes more phage. The cell is destroyed and this is known as lysis. Phages escape and enter and destroy other cells. A drop of phage concentrate on a plate seeded with sensitive bacteria and incubated will show a clear area of lysis.

Phages tend to be active against certain bacterial strains and if a number of different phages are used a pattern of lysis is obtained (Figure 2.5). Phage typing is the commonest method used for typing *Staph. aureus*. A set of numbered phage suspensions are applied to plates seeded with unknown

Table 2.2   Staphylococcal phages

Group I	29	52	52A	79	80	(81)	
Group II	3A	3C	55	71			
Group III	6	42E	47	51	54	75	77
	83A	84	85				
Miscellaneous	94	95	96	88			

types of *Staph. aureus* and after overnight incubation the pattern of lysis is read. Staphylococcal phages are divided into three groups and numbered as shown below in Table 2.2. Group I strains, e.g. 52/80, 29/52A/80, are commonly found in normal noses and can cause boils and septic lesions. Group II strains, especially 71, may cause impetigo. Group III strains, e.g. 6/47/53/54/75, may cause wound infections. However, all phage types can be found in the noses of healthy people.

Phage types are considered to be different if there are two or more major differences, especially if different groups are involved, e.g. 52 is different from 52/52A/79.

It must be realized that phage typing shows differences but similar types are not necessarily related. It is unlikely that a strain 52 isolated in the USA will be related epidemiologically to a similar type isolated in the UK. Many of the staphylococcal strains isolated in recent years, especially MRSA, are non-typable and new phages are being used to differentiate these strains.

Bacteriocins

These are antibiotic-like substances produced by bacteria. As with phages, they are specific to species and usually to strains. Tests are made by growing the unknown strain on a culture plate and recording the inhibition of

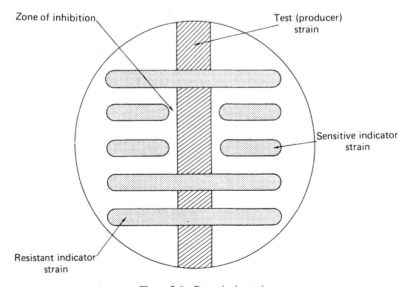

Figure 2.6   Bacteriocin typing

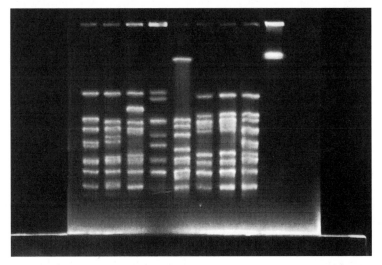

Figure 2.7 Macrorestriction fragments of *Staph. epidermidis* chromosomal DNA treated with the restriction enzyme *sac*II and separated by pulsed-field gel electrophoresis (PFGE). Lanes 1–4 shows isolates from different hip infections and lanes 5–8 show isolates from central venous catheters (gel supplied by Dr AM Livesley and Dr PA Lambert, Aston University, Birmingham)

indicator strains (Figure 2.6). Patterns of inhibition are recorded as in phage typing. The method is sometimes useful for typing *Ps. aeruginosa* or *Klebsiella*, but is often insufficiently discriminatory unless combined with another method. Reproducibility is often poor and the method is now not often used.

Molecular methods of typing

Many organisms causing outbreaks of hospital infection are often non-typable by conventional methods, or no established method is available for typing them, or the strains are similar in type but are of doubtful epidemiological relationship. Conventional methods of typing are also often too slow for rapid identification of outbreak strains and usually have to be carried out in reference laboratories. Molecular methods can often be useful in these instances, particularly as a 'fingerprint' technique for investigating outbreaks in a single department or hospital (Pitt, 1994; Struelens, 1996; Tenover *et al.*, 1997). They usually will not replace existing typing methods for assessing inter-hospital spread or for comparing strains internationally, but it is likely that reproducible national or international molecular typing systems will be developed in the future.

Most of the new methods depend on electrophoretic separation of polypeptides, isoenzymes, plasmids or nucleic acids. Comparisons are made of profiles of 'bands' in a gel or on a membrane (Figure 2.7). These may vary from an analysis of a simple extract of cells on a polyacrylamide gel (PAGE) to more complex DNA or RNA associated molecular techniques.

Plasmid (extrachromosomal DNA) typing involves the extraction of plasmid DNA and the comparison of separated plasmid molecules. This technique is easily carried out, but plasmids may be few in number in some organisms and may occasionally be lost.

Restriction endonuclease activity (REA) is measured from an enzymic digest of plasmid or chromosomal DNA, and is useful for the identification of different genomic strains.

Pulsed-field gel electrophoresis (PFGE) separates large molecules of DNA by use of alternating electric fields. This is one of the most useful techniques, especially for non-phage typable MRSA.

DNA hybridization or gene probing, in which known lengths of DNA are labelled and hybridized with the corresponding DNA from an unknown organism. Probes are used for epidemiological typing and for identifying toxins and antibiotic resistance genes. Ribotyping with an rRNA probe is also useful for subdividing species.

Polymerase chain reaction (PCR) is a system in which the amplification of a single strand of DNA containing a small number of base pairs increases them to over a million in several hours. It is used for the detection of small numbers of organisms in body fluids without growing the organism. It has also been used for detecting genes coding for antibiotic resistance, toxins and virulence factors and for typing, although specificity may not be adequate for routine typing. The method may give a false-positive result due to the presence of contaminating DNA. New methods of molecular typing are continually being developed.

References and further reading

Ayliffe, G.A.J., Collins, B.J. and Lowbury, E.J.L. (1967) Ward floors and other surfaces as reservoirs of hospital infection. *J. Hyg. (Camb.)*, **65**, 515–536.

Caddow, P. (ed.) (1989) *Applied Mirobiology*, London, Scutari Press.

Costerton, J.W., Lewandowski, Z., Caldwell, D.E. *et al.* (1995) Microbial biofilms. *Ann. Rev. Microbiol.*, **49**, 711–745.

Greenwood, D., Slack, R., Petherer, J. (eds) (1992) *Medical Microbiology. A Guide to Microbial Infections, Pathogenesis, Immunity, Laboratory Diagnosis and Control*, 14th edn, Edinburgh, Churchill Livingstone.

Lowbury, E.J.L., Thom, B.T., Lilly, H.A. *et al.* (1970) Sources of infection with *Pseudomonas aeruginosa* in patients with tracheostomy. *J. Med. Microbiol.*, **3**, 39–56.

McGowan, J.E. and Metchcock, B.G. (1996) Basic microbiologic support for hospital epidemiology. *Infect. Cont. Hosp. Epidemiol.*, **17**, 298–303.

Pettit, F. and Lowbury, E.J.L. (1968) Survival of wound pathogens under different environmental conditions. *J. Hyg. (Camb.)*, **66**, 393–406.

Phelps, M., Ayliffe, G.A.J. and Babb, J.R. (1986) An outbreak of candidiasis in a special care baby unit; the use of a resistogram typing method. *J. Hosp. Infect.*, **7**, 13–20.

Pitt, T.L. (1994) Recent developments in typing methods. *PHLS Lab. Digest*, **9**(4), 160–165.

Struelens, M.J. (1996) Laboratory methods in the investigation of outbreaks of hospital-acquired infection. In *Surveillance of Nosocomial Infections* (A.M. Emmersson and G.A.J. Ayliffe, eds), Clin. Infect. Dis., Vol. 3, London, Bailliere Tindall, pp. 267–288.

Tenover, F.C., Arbeit, R.D. and Goering, R.V. (1997) How to select and interpret molecular strain typing methods by epidemiological studies of bacterial infections. A review for health care epidemiologist. *Infect. Cont. Hosp. Epidemiol.*, **18**, 426–448.

Wilson, J. (1995) *Infection Control in Clinical Practice*, London, Bailliere Tindall.

3

Infection and the spread of micro-organisms

Infection

Infection means the deposition of organisms in tissues and their growth with an associated tissue reaction. If the response of the host is slight or nil, this is usually termed 'colonization'. An example is the growth of a strain of *Staphylococcus aureus* in the nose of a healthy person. The staphylococcus grows in the anterior nares without causing any tissue reaction and the person is unaware of being a carrier. Organisms colonize other body sites, e.g. coagulase-negative cocci (*Staphylococcus epidermidis*) grow on normal skin, and *Escherichia coli* is a normal inhabitant of the intestinal tract. *Staph. aureus* and various Gram-negative bacilli are often found on the surface of operation wounds, varicose ulcers or pressure sores without apparently causing any additional tissue damage. Growth of organisms associated with a tissue reaction (i.e. inflammation) is usually referred to as sepsis or clinical infection. A septic wound is usually hot, red and swollen and will eventually produce pus, and bacteriological culture will usually show a heavy growth of the causative organism. A colonized wound may produce a similar growth but the wound will look healthy. For this reason, a wound or other lesion should not be called infected unless there is evidence of tissue damage. Nevertheless, colonization of several patients with the same strain may be an important indication of an organism spreading in a ward or unit. Infection may be inapparent (subclinical) or may show clinical signs (clinical). Organisms may remain in the tissues or body cavities after a clinical infection without causing symptoms. The patient is termed a carrier, but an immunological response to the original infection may remain.

How many organisms are required to cause an infection?

Another major problem is defining an infective dose. Large numbers of *Staph. aureus*, e.g. 100 000 cells (10^5) can be applied to the intact skin without causing a clinical infection and even if this number is injected, an infection may not necessarily occur. However, in the presence of a foreign body, such as a suture, 100 (10^2) organisms may start a clinical infection (Elek and

Conen, 1975). Small numbers of organisms may cause infection if they are able to grow without interference by the body's defences, e.g. in a haematoma. Similarly, large numbers of salmonella, e.g. 1 million (10^6), may be ingested without infection, but if gastric acidity is deficient infection may be caused by small numbers, e.g. 100.

The susceptibility of the host is of major importance and this can rarely be assessed. Factors such as age, sex and pre-existing disease may all be of importance, but are difficult to quantify in terms of susceptibility in an individual. Deficiencies in defence mechanisms can rarely be detected in routine laboratory tests.

Another unknown variable is the virulence of the organism – the ability of the organism to cause infection. Unfortunately no laboratory test is usually available to determine differences in virulence between strains of the organisms causing hospital infection, although tests are available to determine individual virulence factors, e.g. enterotoxins.

For infection to occur, organisms from a source or reservoir must reach a susceptible site in sufficient numbers, which are difficult to define. Should disinfection of the hands or a surface reduce potential pathogens to less than 1000, 100, 10 or to nil? The hands are more important than the floor, as they are more likely to transfer organisms to a susceptible site. For practical purposes it would seem advisable to reduce potential pathogenic organisms on the hands to less than 100 or on a surface to less than 1000. Although it might seem desirable to reduce them to nil, this may require much more effort and be unnecessary to prevent the spread of infection. Removal of all potential pathogens from the skin of an operation site is obviously desirable, but the necessity of removing the normal flora remains uncertain except possibly in certain high-risk operations.

Numbers of organisms in the environment are discussed in later chapters. Removal of all organisms from instruments is obviously much easier than from skin, although complete removal of biofilms from tubing may be difficult. Nevertheless, numbers on surfaces well away from the patient, e.g. on floors, are of minor relevance. A further problem is that organisms may be in clumps or otherwise protected. One skin scale containing 100 staphylococcal cells is more likely to initiate an infection than a scale containing 10, yet both will produce one colony on a settle plate. The distribution is also relevant, e.g. large numbers on the finger-tips are more important than a similar number on the back of the hand.

The spread of micro-organisms

Spread of infection occurs from a source. A source is a site where pathogenic organisms grow and from which they are transmitted and colonize or cause an infection in another site on the same or in another person. Reservoirs are sites in the environment where organisms grow or contaminate, but do not necessarily transmit infection. Removal or destroying a reservoir will not prevent transmission of infection, unless it is also a potential source. Sources are usually infected or colonized patients or staff, or less frequently the inanimate environment.

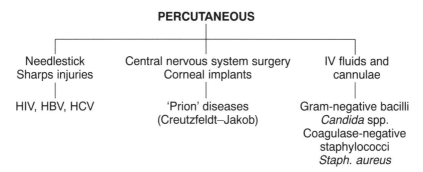

PERCUTANEOUS

Needlestick Sharps injuries	Central nervous system surgery Corneal implants	IV fluids and cannulae
HIV, HBV, HCV	'Prion' diseases (Creutzfeldt–Jakob)	Gram-negative bacilli *Candida* spp. Coagulase-negative staphylococci *Staph. aureus*

Figure 3.1   Transmission of infection – percutaneous routes

The spread of infection from a colonized or infected host or another source depends on the following:

- the numbers of organisms shed from the source
- a route of spread from the source, e.g. air, contact via hands or equipment
- survival of organisms in the environment in sufficient numbers or of sufficient virulence to initiate infection
- a site of entry for the organisms into a new host or another site on the same host
- an ability of the organisms to overcome the host immune system and to multiply in susceptible tissues and initiate an infection.

A risk assessment of likelihood of spread should take into account these factors.

Micro-organisms commonly spread by the airborne route, or by direct or indirect contact, or by the percutaneous or parenteral route. The mode of spread of infection in hospital is rarely certain but apart from respiratory viruses, tubercle bacilli, legionella and occasionally staphylococci, the airborne route is usually a minor one. Airborne transmission from the respiratory tract is usually due to droplet nuclei (5 µm of smaller) which can be dispersed widely without settling. Larger droplets from the respiratory tract settle usually within several feet and are considered to be an extension of contact spread. Common modes of spread and organisms are shown in Figures 3.1, 3.2 and 3.3 and are either endogenous or exogenous. Endogenous infections are acquired from the patient's own bacterial flora and exogenous from other patients or staff (cross-infection) or inanimate sources. In addition to contact and airborne routes, spread may occur by injection of parenteral fluids (Gram-negative bacilli, candida and staphylococci) and blood or body fluids (HBV, HCV and HIV).

In this chapter, we shall mainly consider shedding of organisms and their survival. Heavy dispersal from a source is one of the main factors in the spread of infection (Figure 3.4). Maximal dispersal tends to occur during the acute stage of an infection, e.g. during sneezing and coughing, acute diarrhoea or from discharging wounds or skin surfaces, but, although less likely, transmission can also occur during the later part of the incubation period, from colonized sites, or from post-infection carriage sites.

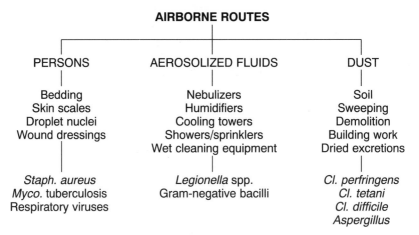

Figure 3.2 Transmission of infection – airborne routes

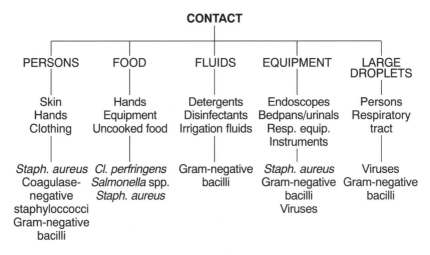

Figure 3.3 Transmission of infection – contact spread

Staphylococcal infection

This organism colonizes the anterior nares in about 20% of healthy individuals, occasionally the perineum and less frequently other areas of skin. Other areas may be contaminated from a carrier site, e.g. the face, neck, hair and hands from a heavy nasal carrier, or the buttocks, abdomen and fingers from a perineal carrier. However, abnormal skin (e.g. eczematous) may be heavily colonized. Staphylococci are rarely shed directly into the air from the nose or mouth during normal breathing or talking, but are mainly shed on skin scales from areas of contaminated skin, e.g. the face or hands. This explains why masks are of little value in preventing the transfer of *Staph. aureus* from staff to patients. A person who sheds large numbers of

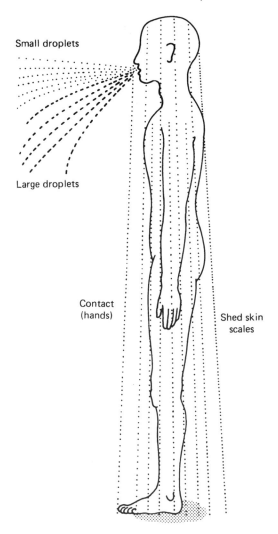

Small droplets

Large droplets

Contact
(hands)

Shed skin
scales

Figure 3.4 Microbial dispersal

Staph. aureus into the air is known as a disperser and is a particular danger in an operating theatre. Dispersers usually have large numbers of staphylococci on the carrier site, e.g. the nose or perineum, and the organisms tend to contaminate other areas of skin in greater numbers than carriers of small numbers (Solberg, 1965).

Dispersal is measured by air-sampling in a small room or plastic chamber while the person concerned carries out some standard exercises or removes clothes. Table 3.1 shows that healthy males tend to disperse more than healthy females, possibly because they shed more skin scales (Ayliffe *et al.*, 1973; Blowers *et al.*, 1973). Male perineal carriers tend to be dispersers and should be looked for in an outbreak in an operating theatre.

Table 3.1   Dispersal of *Staphylococcus aureus* from nasal carriers

	No. of subjects	No. of colonies in 50 ft³ of air		
		0–20	21–50	>50
Females	30	29 (97%)	1 (3%)	0
Males	34	23 (67%)	5 (15%)	6 (18%)

The additional risk of spread of *Staph. aureus* from long hair and beards is often queried. In general, these are only a hazard if the person is a heavy nasal or skin carrier of an epidemic strain. In our experience most of the outbreaks of theatre-acquired infection arise from staff with lesions, e.g. boils, eczema and fungal infections of the groin, although occasionally airborne spread will occur from healthy carriers. In the ward heavy dispersers are usually patients with discharging purulent lesions, bed sores, burns and widespread skin lesions; an eczematous patient colonized with a potential epidemic strain in a surgical ward is a major hazard.

As already described, *Staph. aureus* survives well on drying and can spread by the airborne route, but in the hospital the opportunities for spread by contact are greater. A heavy disperser will contaminate clothing and bedding and will readily contaminate the hands and clothing of attendants (Hambraeus, 1973) Organisms can be transferred to other patients in much greater numbers by contact than in the air. This demonstrates again that handwashing and wearing a protective plastic apron when in contact with an infected patient is much more important than an expensive ventilation system. It should also be remembered that, although staphylococci survive fairly well in a dry environment, they do not grow and gradually die. Numbers of organisms shed into the dry environment decrease within a few days to small numbers, although some survive for months. Airborne contamination of fomites, e.g. curtains and furnishings, and of floors, plays a minor role in the spread of staphylococci and a room left overnight after occupation by a patient infected with staphylococci is unlikely to be responsible for infecting a subsequent patient. Nevertheless, it is still advisable to clean a room thoroughly and change the curtains after occupation by a heavy disperser of a virulent or epidemic strain.

Routine screening of staff in the absence of an outbreak is not of value since it is usually not possible to determine virulent staphylococci from laboratory tests. However, epidemic strains are often resistant to several antibiotics and tend to occur in much larger numbers in the environment than the more sensitive non-epidemic strains. Much more rarely, sensitive or penicillin-resistant strains may spread if dispersed in large numbers, e.g. from a patient with a urinary tract infection, but rarely spread to many patients unless in a neonatal nursery. Endogenous spread of *Staph. aureus* from a carrier site to an operation or traumatic wound during surgery is a common mode of infection. How this occurs remains uncertain as staphylococci can rarely be found on or around the operation site after effective skin disinfection.

Coagulase-negative staphylococci

Coagulase-negative staphylococci are causing an increasing number of infections, particularly following implant surgery, intravascular infusions, in immunosuppressed patients and in neonates. Spread occurs as with *Staph. aureus*, but the organisms are present as residents on all areas of skin and are often more difficult to remove by disinfectants. Airborne spread has been shown to occur from staff in the operating room during implant surgery (Lidwell *et al.*, 1982). Strains may be resistant to several antibiotics, often including gentamicin and methicillin. The problem of differentiating strains, and the large number of different types found on normal skin, make it difficult to define the mode of spread and whether infections are endogenous or exogenous. Although spread can occur in hospital wards, epidemics appear to be uncommon but may not always be recognized.

Streptococccal infections

Viridans and non-haemolytic streptococci are part of the normal flora of the mouth and throat and rarely cause local infections. Viridans-type streptococci can cause endocarditis if they enter the bloodstream of persons with valvular heart disease. Certain strains, e.g *Streptococcus mutans*, are associated with dental caries. *Strep. pyogenes* (Lancefield group A β-haemolytic streptococci) is a cause of tonsillitis, scarlet fever and some cases of puerperal fever, and can cause severe infections of burns and graft failure, infection of operation wounds and skin, e.g cellulitis, erysipelas and very rarely an acute necrotizing fasciitis. Infections tend to be less severe than in the pre-antibiotic era and scarlet fever and erysipelas, which were quite common, are now rarely seen in the developed world. Immunologically associated diseases, rheumatic fever and nephritis are now also rare in the developed world, but still occur in developing countries. The organism appears to be less virulent than in the earlier part of the century, but severe and fatal infections still occur, especially in the elderly, although it has remained sensitive to benzylpenicillin.

The organism can be commonly isolated from the throat of healthy subjects and the mode of spread is mainly by close contact via large droplets or the hands of staff and occasionally in the air in droplet nuclei or on skin scales. Other carriage sites can be associated with cross-infection, e.g. from staff in the operating theatre, and include the skin, anus and vagina. It has also been shown, although now uncommon, that nasal carriers can cause outbreaks of infection. It seems likely that nasal carriers contaminate the face and hands and dispersal occurs on skin scales. The organism can readily be isolated in the air, on bedding and on the floors of wards containing infected patients. However, reducing numbers in the air by oiling blankets and floors was rarely successful in reducing cross-infection in the pre-antibiotic days. It has also been shown that *Strep. pyogenes* in the inanimate environment may lose its virulence. Army recruits issued with blankets contaminated with the organism from infected patients failed to develop infection and contaminated dust blown into the noses of volunteers also failed to infect. However, puerperal fever has been acquired from contaminated shower heads. Although infected burns and widespread skin lesions can cause heavy contamination of the environment including the air, the main route of spread is probably on the hands and clothing of staff.

Other streptococci

Group B streptococci colonize the vagina and rectum of healthy females. Neonates may be infected (meningitis and septicaemia) from the mother during delivery, but cross-infection can occur later in the nursery, presumably on the hands of staff.

Anaerobic streptococci are part of the normal flora of the gastrointestinal tract and can cause endogenous wound and puerperal infections.

Strep. pneumoniae is present in the normal flora of the upper respiratory tract of healthy persons and most cases of pneumococcal pneumonia are endogenous in origin. However, the emergence of resistance to antibiotics, particularly to penicillin, has further shown that cross-infection can occur.

Enterococci (Enterococcus faecalis and faecium), Group D streptococci

Enterococci have become increasingly important as a cause of hospital infection in recent years and strains resistant to β lactams, aminoglycosides and vancomycin (VRE) are increasingly causing outbreaks of infection, particularly in intensive care and other high-risk units. These VRE strains (sometimes referred to as glycopeptide resistant (GRE)) may have been selected by the increasing use of vancomycin for treating MRSA infections. Vancomycin resistance has been transferred from enterococci to *Staph. aureus in vitro* and the possible risk of this occurring in strains in hospitals as well as difficulties in treating infections has increased the need to prevent spread. Low-level resistance of *Staph. aureus* to vancomycin has recently been described in Japan

Enterococci are part of the normal flora of the intestinal tract and may also be isolated from the vagina, skin and mouth. They are a cause of urinary tract, wound, biliary tract and intravenous-catheter-related infection, colonization of pressure sores and rarely endocarditis. They survive well in the dry environment and are more resistant to heat than most non-sporing organisms. Occasional strains show resistance to commonly recommended moist heat disinfection temperatures, i.e. 70°C for 3 min, but most strains are still killed at this temperature and have remained sensitive under practical conditions to the usual chemical disinfectants (Bradley and Fraise, 1996). They can be present in large numbers in the environment, particularly in association with patients with diarrhoea from any cause, and have been isolated from ward surfaces, toilets, commodes, the chamber of bedpan washers, electronic rectal probes and fluidized microsphere beds. They are generally of low pathogenicity and spread is mainly endogenous from the faeces, but spread can occur also on the hands of staff or on contaminated equipment. The role of the inanimate environment in outbreaks remains uncertain.

Gastrointestinal infections

These are spread from the faeces and sometimes vomit of an infected or colonized person or from contaminated food. In general, a heavy dose of organisms is required unless gastric acid is absent. During the acute stages of dysentery, food poisoning or gastroenteritis caused by pathogenic strains of *E. coli* (enteropathogenic, enterotoxigenic, verotoxigenic (strain 0157), enteroinvasive) or salmonellae, large numbers of organisms are shed in the faeces. In infants or incontinent patients this may be associated with heavy environmental contamination. The organisms tend to die rapidly on drying, but if the initial numbers shed are very high some will survive and may even be transferred by the airborne route. This has been reported for enteropathogenic *E. coli* and salmonellae. However, this is rare and in our investigations, environmental sampling in rooms of infected patients have so far yielded few organisms except from bedding in immediate contact with the patient. In recent years, outbreaks of rotavirus and small round virus infections have been increasingly reported in infant nurseries and in geriatric establishments. Large numbers of virus particles are found in the faeces and spread is again probably associated with heavy environmental contamination and dispersal.

Sometimes contaminated equipment has been responsible for the spread of enteropathogens, e.g. resuscitation equipment in neonates, but the main mode of spread is on the hands, or possibly the clothing of attendants.

After the acute stages of diarrhoeal infections have passed, the numbers of organisms in the faeces decrease and transmission is uncommon in adults. Infection can occur from carriers but provided care is taken with personal hygiene the risk is small. Spread from food is described in Chapter 14.

Clostridium difficile is a spore-forming organism frequently found in the normal intestinal tract. It produces two main toxins, A and B. The toxins cause diseases ranging from a mild antibiotic-associated diarrhoea to a severe pseudomembranous colitis, particularly in the elderly and less frequently in neonates. It is selected by antibiotic therapy which includes clindamycin, and to a lesser extent penicillins and cephalosporins, erythromycin or quinolones. It survives well in the environment. Profuse diarrhoea can cause considerable environmental contamination, e.g. of bedding, floors, toilets and bedpans. Incontinent patients are a particular hazard. Transmission is probably mainly on the hands or clothing of staff, but transfer on equipment, such as sigmoidoscopes or rectal thermometers, is possible.

The organism is resistant to commonly used environmental disinfectants and complete removal from the environment is difficult, but the role of the environment in spread of infection is uncertain. Thorough washing of surfaces is usually recommended and should be effective, but addition of chlorine-releasing agents is sometimes recommended. The organism is rapidly killed by 2% glutaraldehyde (5–10 min), but this is not suitable for environmental use.

Other Gram-negative bacillary infections

Most hospital infections caused by Gram-negative bacilli are endogenous in origin. Transfer is directly to the wound from the operation site in the intestinal tract or via the urethra to the urinary tract. Cross-infection is particularly likely in intensive care units, urological wards and special-care baby units. Transmission is mainly on the hands of staff but spread can occur from contaminated equipment, e.g. wash bowls, urinals, bedpans, respiratory equipment (Lowbury *et al.*, 1970). Since Gram-negative bacilli die rapidly on drying, airborne spread is rare. It has been reported from nebulizers contaminated with *Pseudomonas aeruginosa*. Spread by aerosols from contaminated cleaning equipment is a possibility, but reports of wounds infected from this source are usually unconvincing. Airborne spread is possible when burns dressings are changed. Presumably this is again an instance of dispersal of very large numbers of which some survive in the air and the dry environment. Gram-negative bacilli can rarely be isolated in the air of burns or intensive care wards and this mode of spread must be rare. *Acinetobacter* spp. survive well in the environment and are sometimes part of the resident skin flora. They can spread in the air. (*Legionella* see below.)

Respiratory infections

Viral infections involving the upper respiratory tract spread in the air as droplet nuclei, or more usually by close contact with large droplets (Breuer and Jeffries, 1990), although evidence suggests that spread on the hands may be important. Influenza virus can survive for some hours on inanimate surfaces. It is likely that both airborne large droplets and contact play a role in the spread of these viruses. Heavy dispersers are again the main sources and cross-infection is most likely in the late incubation period or early days of an infection when virus concentrations are highest. As the concentration falls, the risks of transmission decrease. Some infections are particularly likely to spread in the air, e.g. chicken-pox and to a lesser extent measles. It is likely that the dose required to initiate infection in these diseases is low in susceptible individuals. Respiratory syncytial virus survives reasonably well in the environment, e.g. in nasal secretions the virus survives on the skin for half an hour, on porous surfaces for 1 h and up to 7 h on non-porous surfaces. Spread is mainly by close contact. It is spread on the hands of staff and can infect staff, causing a prolongation of the outbreak. Outbreaks are usually in paediatric wards initiated by admissions from the community. Herpes simplex virus will also survive on surfaces for several days but spread is mainly by direct contact with the lesion.

Tuberculosis is the other important infection which spreads in the air. The patient with an open lesion of the lung and large numbers of organisms in the sputum, i.e. the heavy disperser, is the main hazard and small particles, i.e. droplet nuclei, must reach the alveoli to initiate a pulmonary infection (Bloom, 1994). Spread from other types of tuberculosis, e.g. urinary tract, is unlikely as numbers tend to be smaller and the opportunity to reach a susceptible site in the respiratory tract of another person is minimal.

Legionnaires' disease is a type of pneumonia caused by *Legionella pneumophila*, or occasionally other species. The organism can be isolated from soil, surface water and water supplies. Eradication is therefore difficult (see Chapter 8). The numbers increase in biofilms formed in water pipes (see page 23), particularly in association with static water. Survival of ingested organisms in amoebae present in the biofilm may protect them from the low concentrations of chemicals present in water supplies. Spread occurs mainly from small droplets (5 μm in diameter) produced by air-conditioning cooling towers in hospitals and hotels. Outbreaks, particularly in immunosuppressed patients, have arisen from calorifiers in hot water systems, dead legs in water systems and infrequently from showers. The mode of transmission is not always clear, but person-to-person spread has not been reported.

Parenteral spread

The problems of growth of organisms in intravenous fluids has been discussed in Chapter 2. The main hazard is from Gram-negative bacilli growing to large numbers in the fluid, and every effort should be made to prevent this, by not leaving containers exposed for too long at room temperature after opening, and keeping blood at 4°C. A heavy growth of organisms in intravenous fluids is now rare, but small numbers of skin organisms, e.g. coagulase-negative staphylococci, may be inoculated with additives. Although these may not grow in the fluids, they may colonize the internal surface of the catheter. The sources of catheter-related infection are mainly the skin around the insertion site or the hands of staff when changing the administration set or introducing additives. *Candida* spp. will also grow well in some fluids used for total parenteral nutrition.

Bloodborne spread of viruses

Hepatitis B has been a problem in recent years, particularly since the outbreaks in dialysis units in the early 1970s. Spread in hospital is mainly by needle stick or other sharp instrument injuries and is now rarely acquired from transfusion blood or blood products. The risk from an injury from a contaminated syringe and needle has been assessed at 20%. Although the virus can be isolated from secretions, spread from these appear to be rare. The risk of spread is greater from patients with acute infection when the virus concentration in the blood is high. Virus concentration may also be high in patients with renal failure. Infectivity is greater if the e-antigen can be detected in blood. Patients have rarely been infected from e-antigen-positive surgeons. This has occurred in deep abdominal surgery, e.g. in pelvic operations, where a sharps injury to the surgeon is more likely. Spread can occur from carriers of surface antigen (HBsAg), but the risks are much less. The reduction in the incidence of hospital-acquired infection has been mainly due to increased care in dealing with infected patients and carriers, screening of blood for transfusion and immunization of staff at risk. Improved hygienic techniques and care in handling blood and needles has considerably reduced the hazards in surgery and in labour wards. Acquisition in laboratories is now rare. Airborne or droplet spread is not a hazard, although it is possible that infection could occur via the conjunctiva if splashing occurs. Wearing of spectacles when operating on carriers is probably worth while, although the evidence for infection via this route suggests that in practice it is rare. Administration of vaccine to all high-risk groups should further reduce risks of infection.

Hepatitis C is also transferred mainly in blood, and most hospital-acquired cases have arisen from blood or blood products. The incidence should be reduced as all transfusion blood in the UK is now screened. The risk of spread from a syringe needle from an infected patient appears to be less than HBV but greater than HIV. This risk varies with the incidence of normal carriage in the community, but is probably about 1–2%. Transmission has been reported in several patients on an operation list and respiratory equipment was suggested as a possible source but this would seem to be unlikely. Prevention of spread is as for HBV but a vaccine is not yet available.

The human immunodeficiency virus (HIV) causes considerable anxiety in health care workers, although there is little evidence of transfer to staff. It is transferred mainly by sexual intercourse, by blood transfusion or blood products. A small number of infections in health care workers have occurred from injuries from needles used on infected patients. However, many contaminated needle stick injuries have occurred in health care workers throughout the world without transferring infection, whereas hepatitis B virus (HBV) has often been transferred by this route. It seems likely that the smaller number of HIV than HB virions in the blood of infected patients considerably decreases the chance of infection. Several infections have also been reported from contamination of damaged skin by infected blood. HIV has been isolated from most body fluids, including saliva, but evidence available suggests that spread from these fluids in the absence of a traumatic injury is unlikely. A report from Italian workers in 1993, which includes other prospective studies as well as their own, stated that there was evidence of 9/3628 (0.25%) seroconversions from percutaneous exposures and 1/1107 (0.09%) from mucous membrane exposures (Ippolito *et al.*, 1993). The virus will survive for some days in exudate on surfaces, but indirect spread or airborne spread has not been reported. The virus is unstable and is more readily inactivated by chemical agents such as glutaraldehyde, hypochlorites, 70% ethanol, some detergents and heat than the hepatitis B virus. The present routine tests available are for antibody which often appears several months after infection. This indicates that recently infected patients may not be detectable by HIV antibody tests. There is little evidence of surgeons or dentists acquiring an infection while operating on an infected patient, but one or two laboratory staff working with the virus have been infected. Spread has rarely been reported from a member of the health care staff to a patient. There has been one report on the spread of infection from an infected dentist to several patients. The mechanism of spread is unknown. The risk of spread is increased by deep injury, visible blood on the device, or a device introduced directly into a blood vessel, particularly if blood is injected. An infected mother may transfer infection to her baby during birth, but transfer by contact after birth is less likely. The virus has been isolated in breast milk, and occasionally spreads by this route (Working Party Report, 1997).

Prion diseases

Creutzfeldt–Jakob disease is one of a series of rare transmisible diseases of man and animals with a long incubation period, e.g. 10–20 years in man, and characterized by progressive dementia. It is believed to be caused by prions (see pages 25 and 166). It occurs mainly in the elderly, but cases have been reported in younger people (new variant CJD). Transmission has occurred from contaminated human pituitary growth hormone and spread has been reported from corneal transplants and surgical instruments. It is also probable that transmission occurs to humans from BSE in cows. The main risk of spread is from central nervous system tissues, although care in handling blood is usually suggested (Advisory Group Committee on Dangerous Pathogens, and Spongiform Encephalopathy Advisory Committee, 1998).

References and further reading

Advisory Committee on Dangerous Pathogens and Spongiform Encephalopathy Advisory Committee (1998) *Transmissable Spongiform Agents: safe working conditions and the prevention of infection*, London, HMSO.

Ayliffe, G.A.J. and Lowbury, E.J.L. (1982) Airborne infection in hospital. *J. Hosp. Infect.*, **3**, 217–240.

Ayliffe, G.A.J., Babb, J.R., and Collins, B.J. (1973) Dispersal and skin carriage in healthy male and female subjects and patients with skin disease. In *Airborne Transmission and Airborne Infection* (J.F.Ph. Hers and K.C. Winkler, eds), Utrecht, Oesthoek Publishing Co., pp. 435–437.

Benenson, A.S., (1995) *Control of Communicable Diseases in Man*, 16th edn, New York, American Public Health Association.

Bloom, B.R. (1994) *Tuberculosis, Pathogenesis, Protection and Control*, Washington, ASM Press.

Blowers, R., Hill, J. and Howell, A. (1973) Shedding of *Staphylococcus aureus* by human carriers. In *Airborne Transmission and Airborne Infection* (J.F.Ph. Hers and K.C. Winkler, eds), Utrecht, Oesthoek Publishing Co., pp. 432–434.

Bradley, C.R. and Fraise, A.P. (1996) Heat and chemical resistance of enterococci. *J. Hosp. Infect.* **34**, 191–196.

Breuer, J., and Jeffries, D.J. (1990) Control of virus infections in hospital. *J. Hosp. Infect.*, **16**, 191–221.

Elek, S.D. and Conen, P.E. (1975) The virulence of *Staphylococcus pyogenes* for man. A study of the problems of wound infection. *Br. J. Exp. Path.*, **38**, 573–586.

Hambraeus, A., (1973) Transfer of *Staph. aureus* via nurses' uniforms. *J. Hyg. (Camb.)*, **71**, 799–814.

Ippolito, G., Puro, V., de Carli, G. and the Italian Study Group on occupational risk of HIV infection (1993) The risk of occupational human immunodeficiency virus infection in healthcare workers. *Arch. Int. Med.*, **153**, 1451–1458.

Lidwell, O.M., Lowbury, E.J.L., Whyte, W. *et al.* (1982) Effect of ultraclean air in operating rooms on deep sepsis in the joint after total hip or knee replacement: a randomized study. *Br. Med. J.*, **295**, 10–14.

Lowbury. E.J.L., Thom, B.T., Lilly, H.A. *et al.* (1970) Sources of infection with *Pseudomonas aeruginosa* in patients with tracheostomy. *J. Med. Microbiol.*, **3**, 39–56.

Mayhall, C.G. (ed.) (1996) *Hospital Epidemiology and Infection Control*, Baltimore, Williams and Wilkins.

Reybrouck, G. (1983) Role of the hands in the spread of nosocomial infection. *J. Hosp. Infect.*, **4**, 103–110.

Solberg, C.O. (1965) A study of carriers of *Staphylococcus aureus. Acta Med Scand*, **178**, (suppl. 436).

Working Party Report (1997) *HIV Infection in Maternity Care and Gynaecology*, London, Royal College of Obstetricians and Gynacologists, RCOG Press.

4

Outbreaks of infection and infectious diseases: investigation and action

The definition of an outbreak is often difficult, but for practical purposes in hospital it can be considered as two or more epidemiologically related infections caused by an organism of the same type. The main problem is to identify common organisms as being similar in type as rapidly as possible (see Chapter 2). *E. coli* is a common cause of urinary tract infection and most infections due to sensitive strains are endogenous in origin. Several endogenous infections may occur in catheterized patients in a ward at the same time and a suitable rapid typing method is not usually available, although biotyping may sometimes be useful. If the strains are resistant to several antibiotics or one unusual antibiotic, such as gentamicin, cross-infection is a more likely explanation. Similarly, penicillin-resistant strains of *Staph. aureus* are commonly present in the nose of healthy carriers, and phage typing is necessary to determine whether strains are indistinguishable. Even then, certain types are common and could occur by chance in several patients or staff in a ward at the same time. Several infections caused by methicillin- or gentamicin-resistant strains in a ward are suggestive of cross-infection and phage typing is less important, although there is some evidence from molecular typing that they are sometimes different types. If the causative organisms are not commonly part of the normal flora, e.g. *Salmonella typhimurium*, two infections in one ward are likely to be an outbreak. This applies to a lesser extent to β-haemolytic streptococci which may be part of the normal flora, but typing of strains is preferable although it is unwise to await results before taking action. Epidemiological relationships are of importance. Wound infections caused by a similar type of *Staph. aureus* in three different wards may have a common origin in one operating theatre. However, if no connection can be found, the finding of the same strains in different wards is probably of no significance. There are also situations in which one infection can be an indication for action. An infection occurring in a patient who has been in hospital for longer than the incubation period suggests a source in the hospital. A case of typhoid fever in a patient who has been in hospital for 4 weeks suggests a carrier should be sought.

The action taken varies with circumstances. Two minor staphylococcal infections caused by the same penicillin-resistant type may not be sufficient to take immediate action, but the situation should be carefully watched. If the two strains are gentamicin- and methicillin-resistant (or even if there is only one such strain in a high-risk unit, e.g. intensive care) immediate action may be indicated. Immediate action is sometimes needed if only one case, e.g. diphtheria, is identified in the hospital, but a single case of gastroenteritis may only require isolation and clinical surveillance of other patients. Screening of contacts is not usually required unless further cases occur.

For some organisms spreading mainly by colonizing patients, an epidemic strain may be considered as an organism causing infection or colonization involving more than one ward or more than one hospital. A highly epidemic strain is likely to involve a number of hospitals.

Identification of the outbreak

The system of surveillance should detect potential outbreaks as quickly as possible. Ward staff should be encouraged to send samples to the laboratory from all suspected infections. The laboratory staff should save certain reports for inspection by the ICN and should inform the microbiologist of any evidence suggesting a potential outbreak. Reports of the following should be inspected and 'Alert' organisms should be flagged on a report form or a computer:

- all wounds and bacteraemias
- all infections from the special-care baby unit, intensive care, paediatric, other high-risk areas and communicable diseases
- all *Pseudomonas aeruginosa*, Group A haemolytic streptococci, *Salmonella, Shigella*, enteropathogenic *E. coli*, rotavirus, *Mycobacterium tuberculosis*
- highly resistant strains of *Staph. aureus*, or strains resistant to methicillin, fusidic acid or gentamicin, and highly resistant Gram-negative bacilli (or resistant to gentamicin and other aminoglycosides or third-generation cephalosporins or quinolones).

The ward staff (medical and nursing) should also be encouraged to inform The Infection Control Team if infections are occurring in a ward; occasionally microbiological samples or reports are not immediately available, e.g. from a deep wound, or from a patient admitted with diarrhoea in the maternity department.

The decision to keep long-term records is difficult, but it is advisable to keep some (e.g. as above) so that related infections occurring sporadically (e.g. one per week or one every few weeks in one ward) can be recognized. A card index (e.g. Kardex) system with a page for each ward or unit is a convenient method. Computerized records are increasingly being used to identify a predetermined level of infection or to detect a specific organism. It is important that the information is regularly reviewed by the ICT.

Assessment

On visiting the ward, the ICN or ICD will determine the following:

1. Are the infections genuine or are the sites only colonized? Colonization may be an indication of a spreading organism, e.g. methicillin-resistant *Staph. aureus* in several pressure sores.

2.   Are the infections hospital-acquired?
3.   Are they likely to spread?
4.   Is there any evidence of existing cross-infection?

A standard record or form will help to answer these questions. The following should be recorded if an outbreak of wound infection is suspected: ward or department; name, age, sex and hospital number of the patients involved; date of admission; date of onset; date and type of operation; whether the operation site was drained; the time relationship of infection to ward dressings; operating theatre and surgeon; position of patient on operating list; organisms isolated and antibiotic sensitivity patterns; position of patient in ward; antibiotics given.

This information may be sufficient to make an immediate decision without further microbiology tests. For instance, if there are three infections due to different organisms, it is not an outbreak (although there may still be a need to investigate aseptic techniques). A deep infection in an undrained wound was probably acquired in the operating theatre. However, at this stage it may be necessary to decide on the need for further studies, e.g. nose swabs from staff, air-sampling or sampling of equipment. It may also be necessary to arrange for immediate isolation of certain patients, e.g. with a salmonella infection in a maternity unit. Comparison of infected and non-infected patients with similar underlying conditions (matched controls) may provide evidence of factors common to the infected patients, e.g. catheterization. The following should be considered when an outbreak occurs or a case of communicable disease is found in a ward:

1.   Isolation of infected patients.
2.   The need for convening the Major Outbreaks Committee (see below).
3.   Prevention of movement of staff and patients to other wards.
4.   Non-admission of new patients, unless immune.
5.   Sending home as many patients as possible.
6.   Administration of immune serum to highly susceptible patients, e.g. leukaemics exposed to chicken-pox.
7.   Treatment of close contacts, e.g. of diphtheria or meningococcal meningitis.
8.   Informing administration (general, nursing and medical) and notifying public health authorities, e.g. the CDCC.
9.   Introduction of new measures or improving existing procedures, e.g. alcohol disinfection of hands.
10. Closure of wards or introduction of cohort system.
11. Sampling of contacts and environment.

The measures required will obviously have to be decided for each situation and occasionally some risks may be necessary and must be decided on probabilities. The closure of a ward and sampling faeces of all patients and staff when a single case of typhoid fever is recognized on a surgical ward is unnecessary. Typhoid rarely spreads from person to person, but it obviously can. Nevertheless, the risk is so small that closing down an important service should not be necessary. A balance of risks and benefits is required.

It is necessary to keep everyone informed and all movements of patients should be decided with the co-operation of the relevant clinician who has the ultimate responsibility for his patients.

Major outbreaks or infection problems requiring unusual measures

These are difficult to define but usually consist of a large number of infections, e.g. *Salmonella, Legionella*, requiring additional facilities, materials or major staff changes. Examples include: closing of wards; opening a special isolation ward; more nursing, medical or domestic staff; more linen or CSSD materials; assistance from other hospitals, specialist laboratories or the Communicable Disease Surveillance Centre (CDSC) in the UK. A single case of a particularly hazardous disease, e.g. Lassa fever or diphtheria, or an outbreak involving fatal cases or community involvement, may all require special action.

The Major Outbreaks Committee should be convened by the ICD, supported by a senior administrator and the CCDC. It should also include a senior member of the medical staff, e.g. the Medical Director, the nursing staff, e.g. the Executive Nurse Director, the microbiologist, infection control nurses, occupational health doctor and/or nurse, Director of Public Health and an infectious diseases physician if available.

The ICD or CCDC should co-ordinate the investigations and procedures. This will usually be the responsibility of the ICD in hospital or the CCDC if the community is involved, although the CCDC has overall responsibility for the control of communicable diseases in the hospital and the community.

The functions of the committee are:

- to ensure continuing clinical care of infected patients
- to assess resource implications, e.g. staff and materials, and to make suitable arrangements for adequate provision of these
- to agree and co-ordinate policy decisions on investigations and control of outbreak
- to nominate a person for providing information to the media
- to notify Regional Epidemiologist, Department of Health, Communicable Surveillance Centre (CDSC) and other hospitals in the area – this will usually be the responsibility of the CCDC
- to arrange for communication of information on the outbreak to relevant hospital staff, e.g. pharmacy, domestic services, laundry, Sterile Services and supplies, and to visitors and relatives
- to define the end of the outbreak and prepare a written report, including lessons learnt.

In an outbreak where few additional resources are required and the situation can be handled locally, the ICT will remain responsible, but information on progress should be regularly supplied to the administration, medical and nursing staff and the CCDC who may attend meetings of the team. A person should still be nominated to provide information to the media.

Outbreaks of surgical infection with *Staph. aureus*

The following information is useful when considering an outbreak of staphylococcal wound infection:

- Infection with antibiotic-sensitive organisms or strains resistant to penicillin only is likely to be endogenous in origin or acquired in the operating theatre. Multi-resistant strains are usually ward-acquired. However, multi-resistant strains may be acquired before operation, particularly if the length of stay before operation is prolonged and then the infection appears to be endogenous although it was really hospital-acquired.
- Sources are human, often with lesions, and are usually heavy dispersers. Healthy males are more likely to be dispersers and perineal carriers than females. Look for causes which might not be reported, e.g. pressure sores or rashes, particularly of the groin.
- The dry environment is not a major source or route of spread.
- Undrained wounds seal in 1–2 days and infection acquired in the ward is then unlikely, unless the wound has failed to heal.

Infections of theatre origin

Theatre infection is suspected if it is deep and in an undrained, clean, dry wound, or if an infection occurs before any ward dressing is carried out. Infection in drained wounds can originate either in the ward or in the theatre. Similar strains causing infections in different wards, but operated on by the same surgical team, are good evidence of theatre-acquired infection. Visit the theatre and find out which members of staff were present at the operations subsequently infected, and whether any of them has an infected lesion (or non-infected skin lesion, e.g. eczema). The source may be determined at this time with very little disturbance to staff or without much additional microbiology.

If this fails, take nose swabs from all staff. If all are negative, sample the air during an operation performed by the suspect team, or sample the theatre floor with contact plates at the end of the operation for screening.

If the organism is resistant to an antibiotic other than penicillin, it may be usefully incorporated into the culture media.

Sampling of the floors of the changing rooms may also be useful if the source is not identified by other means.

If no nasal carrier of the epidemic strain is found, but it is present in the environment, repeat nasal swabs and sample fingers of staff. If this fails, take perineal swabs and examine all staff for lesions. However, if noses and environment are both negative, continue close surveillance and repeat sampling if infections continue, as some healthy carriers only disperse intermittently and for short periods.

An example of an outbreak

A summary of four infections is shown in Table 4.1. An infection of a herniorrhaphy or a varicose vein operation is likely to be theatre-acquired, and two different wards are involved. Infections occurred in Theatre 2 and the anaesthetist is a primary suspect. If he is not a carrier of the epidemic strain, the staff and environment of Theatre 2 should be examined. Although a member of the scrubbed staff is the most likely source, others in the theatre at the time of the operation may be the source.

Table 4.1   Infections due to penicillin-resistant *Staphylococcus aureus* (phage type 52, 52A, 79)

Infected operation	Operating theatre	Ward	Surgeon	Anaesthetist
Hernia	2	4	Mr A	Dr B
Cholecystectomy	2	1	Mr C	Dr B
Hernia	2	4	Mr A	Dr B
Varicose veins	2	1	Mr A	Dr B

Treatment of a staphylococcal carrier on the staff

This will only be required if the staff member is carrying a strain which is known to be causing infections or is an epidemic strain in the hospital and eradication procedures are in progress. Staff carriers should not be routinely treated.

In the example described above, Dr B is the probable source of the wound infections and this can be confirmed with a nasal swab. If positive, samples should also be taken from the groin/perineum and any lesion. If nasal carriage is confirmed, mupirocin nasal cream 2% should be applied to the anterior nares 3 times a day for 5–7 days. Irrespective of whether the subject is also a skin carrier or has a lesion, an antiseptic should be applied to the skin as contamination of the adjacent skin is likely from the existing carriage site. A daily bath or shower should be taken using an antiseptic detergent (chlorhexidine, triclosan, povidone-iodine or hexachlorophane) for 1 week. The antiseptic should be applied directly to the skin after wetting and before rinsing, paying particular attention to possible carriage sites, e.g. face and bathing trunk area. The hair should be washed with an antiseptic shampoo (e.g. cetrimide) twice during the week followed by a conditioner. Positive sites should be sampled 2 days and 2 weeks after completing a course of treatment. If the staff member is only a nasal carrier, he/she may return to work after 2 days' treatment, with mupirocin. If there is a colonized lesion, the staff member should stay off duty until the organism is removed from the lesion and preferably the lesion is healed. If the lesion is small, it may be possible to occlude it with an impermeable dressing. Small lesions can also be treated with an appropriate mupirocin preparation for up to 7 days. Not more than 2 courses of mupirocin should be given either for treating nasal carriage or a lesion.

If the colonizing strain is mupirocin resistant, or mupirocin-resistant strains are present in the hospital, or two courses of mupirocin have failed to eradicate the strain, it may be advisable to treat carriers with an alternative preparation, e.g. Naseptin (neomycin and chlorhexidine), if the strain is neomycin sensitive, or chlorhexidine cream 1–2%, or a bacitracin cream if available, 4 times a day for a week. This and the antiseptic bathing can be continued for several months if initial treatment has failed. If the antiseptic is causing skin irritation, the antiseptic should be changed or discontinued. Clean clothing and bedding should be used at the end of each course of treatment.

The following should also be considered if treatment fails;

- Sampling of other sites, e.g. throat, rectum or vagina.

- Systemic treatment, e.g. combinations of oral rifampicin and ciprofloxacin, or fusidic acid or erythromycin, for 1 week if the organism is sensitive to both agents. Side effects can occur with these agents, especially with rifampicin and fusidic acid, and careful observation is required during treatment. Topical preparations of agents likely to be used systemically, e.g. vancomycin, fusidic acid, cotrimoxazole, ciprofloxacin and gentamicin, should be avoided if possible, as emergence of resistance is possible.
- Sampling other members of the family should be considered if rapid recurrence of colonization with the same strain occurs.
- A ventilated, bacteria impermeable suit for use by a colonized surgeon during an operation may be effective in reducing dispersal, although this has not been validated in practice.

Outbreaks in the surgical ward (i.e. two or more cases)

Infected patients are the main sources (Figure 4.1).

Investigation
Nose swabs are taken from patients, and swabs are taken from all wounds, lesions, intravenous and urinary catheter sites and sputum if available. Dispersers may be identified by exposing settle plates, by sampling floors or preferably by sweep or contact plates of bedding. If the epidemic strain is resistant to an antibiotic other than penicillin it can be incorporated into the culture media. Although staff carriers can transmit strains in a ward, this is unusual and staff carriers are usually the victims. However, if the outbreak continues consider taking nasal swabs from the staff and perineal/groin swabs and throat swabs from patients in addition to nasal swabs.

Action
Patients with infected lesions should be isolated or sent home and dispersers should be given a priority for isolation. Outbreaks often cease when the main disperser has been removed. Nasal carriers of the epidemic strain should be treated. This applies also to staff, although they are more often victims than causes. Other measures include the use of antiseptic detergents or 70% alcohol for handwashing or disinfection by staff. Antiseptics, e.g. povidone-iodine, chlorhexidine, triclosan or hexachlorophane (not suitable for babies), should be used for bathing, showering or bedbaths routinely.

If the epidemic continues, nasal prophylaxis of all patients and staff should be considered. Wounds (infected or liable to infection) can often be sealed with an adhesive water-vapour-permeable plastic sheet (e.g. Opsite). or covered with an antiseptic-impregnated dressing. Avoid use of topical antibiotics to wounds if possible.

Staphylococcal outbreaks in a neonatal ward

Epidemic strains tend to be penicillin resistant only and to colonize the nose, umbilicus and groins of babies. Spread is from baby to baby, usually via the hands of staff and infrequently in the air. A member of staff or mother may introduce the strain initially into the nursery.

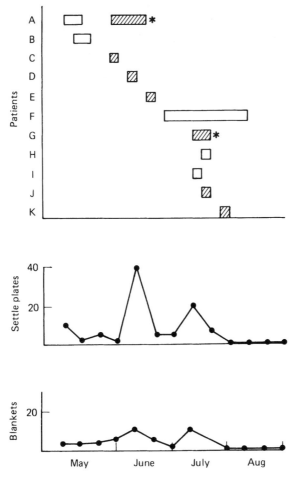

Figure 4.1 Spread of *Staph. aureus* from dispersers A and G with increased air counts and blanket contamination; □, noses; ▨, lesions; *, heavy dispersers

Investigation
Swabs should be taken from noses of nurses and babies and from the umbilicus of babies and any lesion. As in a surgical ward, dispersers may be detected by settle plates or sampling of bedding.

Action
Isolate babies with staphylococcal infection even if there is only one in the ward. If the strain is spreading cohort nursing should be introduced. Carriers should be treated with an antiseptic detergent and nose cream. Hexachlorophane powder 0.3% should be applied to the groins and umbilicus of all babies if this is not in routine use in the unit.

Methicillin-resistant *Staphylococcus aureus* (MRSA)

Methicillin-resistant *Staph. aureus* strains are now present in hospitals of most countries of the world (Wenzel *et al.*, 1991; Ayliffe, 1977). The strains are usually resistant to two or more antibiotics, which may include tetracycline, erythromycin, neomycin, gentamicin, trimethroprim, ciprofloxacin or mupirocin, in addition to the penicillinase-resistant penicillins and cephalosporins. They vary in virulence. Most strains are at least as virulent as methicillin-sensitive strains, although the presence of clinical infection often depends as much on the susceptibility of the host as the virulence of the organism. In general, MRSA are good colonizers of the nose, certain areas of skin, e.g. buttock area in the elderly, and chronic skin lesions. Some strains show a particular propensity to spread and are referred to as epidemic strains (EMRSA). No laboratory test is available to detect either epidemicity or virulence, although typing methods can be helpful during epidemics to identify particular strains. All MRSA must therefore be treated initially as potentially epidemic strains. Outbreaks of MRSA are similar to those of other multi-resistant strains which occurred in hospitals in the 1940s to 1960s. The main differences are that resistance to methicillin causes particular problems in treatment, and some strains appear to be more transmissible than previous epidemic strains. Strains are also more frequently found in the community and are often reintroduced into hospitals on colonized patients without being detected. Methicillin resistance is a good marker and enables MRSA to be more easily detected than methicillin-sensitive epidemic strains, but its importance has been exaggerated by excessive media coverage.

Risk factors for the spread of MRSA

- Elderly patients, especially if confined to bed.
- Prolonged hospital stay.
- Previous antibiotic therapy.
- Presence of chronic skin lesions, e.g. pressure sores, ulcers and dermatitis.
- Invasive procedures, e.g. intravascular and urinary tract catheterization.
- Patients in high infection-risk units, e.g. ICU.
- Tertiary referral hospitals are also particularly at risk.
- Inadequate ward facilities, e.g. large open-plan wards and a shortage of single or isolation rooms, or handwashing facilities.
- Overcrowding, staff shortages, inadequately trained staff.
- Frequent transfers of patients and staff between wards and hospitals.
- Excessive use of antibiotics in a ward.

Investigation and control

The methods are similar to those already described, but EMRSA present particular problems (Report, 1998). They are sometimes present in a number of wards of a hospital without causing many clinical infections and may require excessive efforts to eradicate them. These eradication methods may not be in the interests of optimal patient care and may not be cost effective. However, every effort should be made to control their spread, although some flexibility is required (Spicer, 1984; Ayliffe, 1996). Priorities are suggested if eradication in all wards is not possible and should be based on the following:

- the type of unit, e.g. ICU, orthopaedic and medical, depending on infection risks to patients in the particular unit
- the virulence of the organism (the number and severity of clinical infections) and its potential transmissibility
- the distribution of strains within the hospital
- the admission of the first epidemic strain to a hospital or high-risk unit
- facilities and resources available, e.g. isolation rooms
- laboratory resources.

Procedures

Endemic situation

The definition of endemic is difficult, but if EMRSA are distributed over several wards, or in the community, clinical infections are few and the use of eradication methods are not considered to be cost effective or adequate resources are not available to control the spread, the situation could be described as endemic. It has also been suggested that that if over 10% of laboratory isolates are EMRSA, this would constitute an endemic situation, but this could vary depending on the local distribution of strains.

General control measures

- Good basic hygiene (including cleaning procedures).
- Handwashing with antiseptic detergent or alcohol rub after handling an infected or colonized patient, or his/her immediate surroundings.
- Wearing gloves and a plastic apron for contact with lesions, contaminated dressings or equipment.
- Careful handling of bed linen and clinical waste and transporting in a sealed bag or container as required for 'infected' waste and linen (see Chapters 13 and 15).
- Decontaminate equipment used on an infected or colonized patient, e.g. stethoscope, blood pressure cuff, before use on another patient.
- Audit implementation of control procedures.
- Avoid transfer of patients to other wards. If a visit to another department, e.g. physiotherapy, is essential, instruct staff on precautions necessary.
- If one or more colonized or infected cases are detected in a high-risk ward, eradication measures should be introduced.
- If resources and facilities are available, isolate or cohort nurse infected or colonized patients.

Priorities depending on infection risks

High risk

- Special units containing patients highly susceptible to infection, e.g. ICU, cardiothoracic surgery, intensive care neonatal units, orthopaedic wards, burns units (if organism is virulent), transplant and dialysis units.

- The first epidemic strain admitted to a hospital.
- A highly virulent strain causing severe clinical infections.

Intermediate risk

- High-dependency units, e.g. surgical wards, neonatal wards, urological and gynaecological/obstetric wards.
- Strain predominantly colonizing, but causing some clinical infections in susceptible patients.

Low risk

- Medical wards, acute geriatric and mental health wards.
- Strain mainly colonizing, few clinical infections.

Minimal risk

- Long-term care units. Patients colonized without clinical infection.

Depending on the types of individual patient in a unit and virulence of organism, the *risk category can be changed by the local ICT. During an outbreak all wards in the hospital should be categorized for infection risk.*

Control procedures depending on risk

All wards containing infected or colonized patients should carry out procedures described for endemic infections.

High risk (one or more cases)

- Eradication procedures should be introduced.
- Screen all patients, isolate or cohort nurse all infected or colonized patients. Treat with antiseptic baths and nasal cream or ointment where appropriate (see page 53). If outbreak continues, screen staff and treat if colonized; consider additional screening of patients, e.g. throat, and antiseptic treatment of skin and nasal prophylaxis of all patients in the wards.

Intermediate risk

- Isolate or cohort nurse infected or colonized patients. If more than two cases, consider screening all patients and introduce eradication procedures. If isolation facilities are inadequate, precautions can be decided by a scoring system (e.g. Wilson and Dunn, 1996).

Low risk

- General measures as for endemic infections.

Minimal risk

- No special precautions, apart from good hygienic standards (Report, 1995).

In a hospital or high-risk unit without MRSA, prevention of spread *from first admission* is the highest priority.

Screening of admissions

- All patients previously infected or colonized with MRSA.
- Patients from hospitals with a known MRSA problem (or having been in such a hospital in the past year) unless reported as negative by the transferring hospital.
- Patients from other countries, especially if recently hospitalized.

Admit these patients to a single room or an isolation ward or unit if available until results of screening are available.

Sampling

- Use moistened swabs or contact plates.
- Routine screening of patients in a ward – nose, pressure sores, wounds, eczema or other skin lesions, or sites of invasive devices.
- Routine screening of patients on admission – include perineum/groin.
- Failure to control outbreak – consider sampling throat, perineum/groin, buttock area in bedridden elderly patients, fingers and noses of staff.
- If clinically indicated, sample sputum, urine, faeces, vagina.
- The risk of spread is greatest from a heavy disperser (see page 37), e.g. with infected or colonized lesions, or heavy nasal or skin carriers. Risk from other colonized sites, e.g. throat, vagina or faeces, is unknown. Sampling of bedding with a contact plate may assist in risk assessment of dispersal.
- Sampling for clearance should be made 2 days and 2 weeks after completing treatment. Previous positive sites should be sampled.

Other procedures to be considered

- Patient's notes should be marked so that they can be detected early on readmission or admission to another hospital (and recorded in computer if available).
- Strains may return after clear post-treatment screening samples (at least two sets, preferably three, of negative samples are initially recommended). Recurrence can occur over periods varying from several weeks to up to one year or more.

- Prevent movement of patients or staff as much as possible during an outbreak.
- Check whether agency (i.e. staff employed by an outside agency and moving from ward to ward or hospital to hospital as required) or locums are working or have worked in other hospitals with an MRSA problem. Although staff are not a major source of spread, consider sampling noses of these staff, especially if working in a high-risk unit.
- Inform infection control staff if a patient with MRSA or from an affected ward is transferred to another hospital.
- Develop a communications network between infection control teams for transfer of information on hospitals with an MRSA problem.

Minimal risk areas

Nursing and residential homes are often loath to admit known MRSA carriers (Report, 1995). These patients can block beds in acute wards for long periods at high cost. The staff in these homes must be persuaded by the ICT or CCDC that these carriers do not represent a significant risk to other patients, staff, relatives or visitors. Isolation is not required. Staff should receive some training in basic infection control techniques, e.g. handwashing and aseptic methods, and an explanatory leaflet should be provided (Public Health Environmental Group, 1996).

Ambulance staff should be similarly educated and usually need only to disinfect their hands and change the bedding after transporting MRSA carriers.

Antibiotics

Vancomycin or teicoplanin is usually used for treating severe infections, but other antibiotics may be used if the organism is sensitive. Rifampicin with another agent, e.g. fusidic acid or ciprofloxacin, to reduce the emergence of resistance may be used for treating throat carriers or colonized lesions. However, complications are common with rifampicin and fusidic acid and careful consideration of the necessity to use them is required before treating. Courses of treatment for carriers should usually not be repeated. Colonized or infected patients should be given vancomycin or teicoplanin pro-phylactically if a surgical operation is required. However, a recent report of the isolation of low-level vancomycin-resistant strains from Japan indicates that a possible reconsideration of the use of vancomycin is necessary and use of alternative agents should be considered, if available.

Although previous antibiotic therapy has been associated with MRSA colonization, the role of specific antibiotics in the emergence and spread of MRSA remains uncertain. The more recent increase in the use of cephalosporins has been suggested as a contributory factor, but others, such as the quinolones or trimethroprim, are also possible selecting agents. The rational use of antibiotics, especially limiting the length of courses of treatment and the use of single dose surgical prophylaxis, should be introduced. Restriction of specific agents, such as the cephalosporins, requires further evaluation.

However, *prevention of cross-infection is likely to be the most productive preventative measure.*

Gram-negative bacilli

Most infections are endogenous and infected patients are the main sources in outbreaks, but common-source outbreaks can occur from equipment which comes into close contact with a susceptible site on the patient. Environmental sources are commonly fluids or medical devices. Common organisms causing outbreaks are *Klebsiella/Enterobacter* spp. and *Ps. aeruginosa*, but can include *E. coli, Proteus* spp., other *Pseudomonas* spp., *Serratia marcescens, Acinetobacter* spp. and many other Gram-negative bacilli. Most of these, apart from *E. coli*, can survive well and grow in the moist environment of the ward. Infection has been reported from nebulizers, mechanical ventilators, disinfectant or antiseptic solutions, inadequately sterilized parenteral fluids or saline used at operation, hand creams, shaving brushes, plaster buckets in accident departments, transducers and monitoring equipment and endoscopes. Other possible sources are washing bowls, baths, nail-brushes, soap-dishes and containers, thermometer disinfection fluid, food-mixers, mattresses, urine bottles and bedpans.

The history of the patient may indicate a common source. In an outbreak of *Ps. aeruginosa* in a neurosurgical unit, the organism was only found on the scalp after shaving. Although *Ps. aeruginosa* was widely distributed in the environment, none was the epidemic strain, apart from one strain in a shaving brush (Figure 4.2) which was considered to be the common source.

A similar study in an eye hospital, in which a number of patients lost their sight, showed that the strain was present in saline used to moisten the eye at operation. Phage typing results are shown in Table 4.2.

In neonatal units, a source in the labour ward should be sought if infections are occurring within a few days of birth. Suction equipment is always a possibility. Other moist areas, such as baths, soaps, etc. should be examined.

It is important that infections arising from contaminated intravenous fluids are identified rapidly. The contents of the container should be sampled as soon as possible and the batch number referred to the pharmacy so that suspect containers can be withdrawn from circulation. Unusual organisms,

Table 4.2 Phage patterns of *Ps. aeruginosa* isolated from an eye hospital during an outbreak of infection

Site of isolation	Phage pattern
Bath and sink (bathroom)	7/31/73
Floor, sink, cloth (sluice room)	7/31/73/109/119X
Floor and sink (ward)	7/21/68/119X
Urine bottles + mop and bucket (1)	7/31/73
+ mop and bucket (2)	109/119X
Saline used to irrigate eyes	7/24/68/1214
Eye infections	7/24/68/1214

Phage patterns from environment, apart from saline, differ from those causing infection

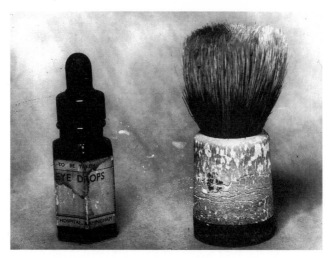

Figure 4.2   Shaving brush and saline contaminated with *Ps. aeruginosa* identified as sources of outbreaks

e.g. *Erwinia*, in a blood culture should alert Infection Control Teams to the possibility and careful surveillance is important, preferably on a national scale. *Acinetobacter* spp. survive well in the dry environment, in the air and on the skin, resembling *Staph. aureus*. Some *Klebsiella* spp. also survive on the skin for longer periods than most Gram-negative bacilli.

Investigation

Information is collected on the patients with infection and should include time of indwelling catheterization, mechanical respiratory ventilation, intravenous cannulation, antibiotic therapy, as well as the usual data on age, length of stay, diagnosis, treatment with steroids, etc. Samples should be collected from all patients where appropriate, e.g. sputa, catheter specimens of urine, wounds, bed sores and other lesions. The indications may be of patient-to-patient cross-infection. It may then be worth while looking at ward techniques, in particular catheter care and respiratory suction. In some instances, a common source may seem likely, and sampling of the relevant item of equipment or fluid is necessary. If the source is still unknown, general environmental sampling should be undertaken. This may bring to light deficiencies not previously recognized, e.g. inadequate disinfection of urine bottles, a bedpan washer/disinfector not working, failure to change tubing attached to a ventilator and topping-up of disinfectant solutions. The hands of the staff should also be sampled. This will demonstrate the importance of handwashing. Typing of strains may be necessary to differentiate between the epidemic strain and others (Lowbury *et al.*, 1970). It must also be realized that equipment may be contaminated from the infected patients and not vice versa; this applies particularly to organisms in mops and sinks.

Action

On completion,of the epidemiological investigation it should be possible to prevent the spread of the organism by good aseptic techniques and adequate decontamination of equipment. An antiseptic detergent or alcoholic solution could be introduced for hand disinfection. If one patient is an obvious source, isolation in a single room may be worthwhile, especially if heavy environmental contamination is likely, although the air is not a major route of spread.

Enterococcal infections

Outbreaks of infection with vancomycin-resistant strains (VRE) are increasingly being reported in intensive care and other high-risk units (Wade, 1995). In the USA and some other countries, spread is now occurring more frequently in other wards. Investigation and control is somewhat similar to that of MRSA, apart from the difference in carriage sites and the lesser role of skin contamination with VRE (see page 42).

Early detection is important. Control consists of isolation of infected cases (and carriers if possible) in a single room or introduction of cohort nursing if there are several cases. Enteric precautions should be implemented. Improved handwashing techniques should be introduced and preferably an alcoholic rub should be used after handling infected patients or their immediate surroundings.

Aseptic techniques should be audited and special attention paid to skin disinfection of catheter sites and care in changing administration sets.

Wounds, including pressure sores, urines of catheterized patients, sputa if available, and sites of invasive devices, especially intravenous catheter sites, should be sampled. If the infections are in an intensive care unit or the outbreak continues, screening of faeces and mouth of all patients should be considered. Spread from a member of staff has been reported, but routine screening of staff faeces is rarely required. The extent of screening of patients and staff and the precautions taken depends on the clinical problem, and priorities may be required.

Treatment of infected patients and carriers is difficult and some strains are resistant to the quinolones and imipenim as well as vancomycin, the aminoglycosides and β-lactams. Carriage of resistant strains may cease after a few weeks without antibiotic therapy, but some may persist for many months.

Items of equipment likely to be contaminated with faeces or urine, e.g. rectal thermometers, bedpans, urinals and sigmoidoscopes, should be adequately decontaminated before reuse. If contamination of the inanimate environment occurs, the area should be thoroughly cleaned and terminal disinfection should be considered, but the value of this as a control of infection measure remains uncertain.

General measures include a reduction in the use of antibiotics, especially cephalosporins, vancomycin and quinolones. The length of time invasive devices are kept in situ should be minimal. Investigation of an outbreak is difficult because of the lack of a routine typing method, but molecular methods such as pulsed-field gel electrophoresis have been used successfully.

Aspergillus infections

Aspergillus spores are present in air, dust and soil (see Chapter 8). Major outbreaks have been associated with the release of large numbers of spores during demolition or renovation of buildings, or from contaminated service ducts in high-risk wards, or from contaminated filters in ventilation systems (Rhame, 1991). Infection is due to the inhalation of spores mainly by immunosuppressed or compromised patients. Units for immunosuppressed patients, especially liver, cardiothoracic and bone marrow transplant, should be fitted with a positive pressure ventilation system providing filtered air capable of removing spores of 2–3 μm diameter. During an outbreak, a mobile air filtration system can be introduced if there is no existing ventilation system. Service ducts and windows should be sealed and surfaces cleaned with a chlorine-releasing compound. Prophylaxis with an antifungal agent should also be considered.

Legionnaires' disease (Fallon, 1994)

Spread is usually in aerosols from air conditioning systems. Infection may also occur from nebulizers or whirlpools, showers or hot water supplies. Person-to-person spread does not occur. The elderly, particularly with pre-existing respiratory disease, heavy smokers or immunosuppressed patients are particularly susceptible. Early detection is important and this is usually based on clinical suspicion. Although the organisms can sometimes be detected in sputum or bronchial washings, diagnosis is often only possible with an antibody test carried out at a later stage of the illness. Isolation of the patient is unnecessary. If the patient has been in hospital for 10 days or more, it is likely to be hospital-acquired. Look for other possible cases, but if none are found further investigation is not necessary. Two or more related cases require investigation. Samples of water (5 litres) should be collected from all possible sources, e.g. water tanks, hot and cold supplies, showers and cooling towers before any control measures are implemented.

Measures include raising the temperature of hot water supplies and additional chlorination (see Chapters 3 and 8). Neither method is entirely satisfactory; temperatures over 55°C are likely to scald elderly people and higher than usual chlorine levels may cause corrosion in the systems. In the event of a major outbreak, convene the Major Outbreaks Committee and consider asking for assistance from local public health laboratories or the Communicable Disease Surveillance Centre (Health and Safety Executive, 1995).

Intestinal infection (*Salmonella, Shigella,* enteropathogenic and toxigenic *E. coli*)

If there is evidence of cross-infection with an intestinal pathogen involving two patients or more, samples of faeces should be collected from all patients and staff with diarrhoea *after* discussion with infection control staff. A history should be taken from infected patients and should include food and drugs taken over the past 48 h. The infected patients should be isolated if possible in a single room with enteric precautions, and always if in a neonatal ward. If isolation is not possible, enteric precautions should still be introduced in the ward, e.g. handwashing after handling patient or surroundings, and care in disposal of faeces, handling bedpans and soiled linen. It may also be possible to nurse all infected patients together in one ward. If the outbreak is large and likely to require additional staff or facilities, the Major Outbreaks Committee should be convened (see page 51).

It may be advisable to close the ward to new admissions and not to transfer staff to other wards. Neonatal wards should always be closed to new admissions if a known pathogen has spread. If an organism is identified, e.g. *Salmonella* or *Shigella*, faeces should be taken from all patients and sampling of staff should be considered; discuss this with the microbiologist before carrying out any mass sampling. The ward can be reopened when diarrhoea has ceased, but preferably when the pathogen can no longer be isolated from faeces. In general, two negative specimens from known cases should be sufficient. However, it may be necessary in some instances to reopen the ward whilst carriers still remain, although they should preferably be isolated.

If it seems likely that food is incriminated, e.g. all cases have eaten the same food, but not matched controls, and infection occurs throughout the hospital at the same time, catering practices and staff require investigation (Chapter 14). Often there will be no evidence of food-borne infection and no pathogen will be isolated. In this case carry out excretion precautions until symptoms cease; avoid admitting new patients, if possible. Check the disinfection of crockery and cutlery.

These infections are often viral in paediatric or geriatric departments and rotavirus may be detected in the faeces, but often a diagnosis is not made. Nevertheless the measures outlined should still be applied.

Outbreaks of diarrhoea, particularly in wards for elderly patients, are frequently caused by *Clostridium difficile* (Cartmill *et al.*, 1994) (see page 43). Other areas where outbreaks have been reported include surgical wards and wards containing immunosuppressed patients, and spread may extend throughout the hospital. Infection is often endogenous, owing to selection by antibiotic therapy in an existing faecal carrier, but several cases in one ward are frequently due to cross-infection. Control of an outbreak involves rapid detection of cases and single room isolation or cohort nursing with enteric precautions. Priority of isolation should be given to those with profuse diarrhoea or who are incontinent. Handwashing of staff should be by removal with soap and water as the organisms are resistant to antiseptics.

Routine screening of faeces may be undertaken during an outbreak, but a decision should be made on what to do with carriers before embarking on a screening programme; 30% or more patients may be carriers of the epidemic strain. Staff are sometimes carriers, but rarely show signs of clinical infection and are usually victims rather than causes of outbreaks.

Spread on equipment such as rectal thermometers has been reported, but sigmoidoscopes, bedpans, toilets and linen are potential sources and should be handled carefully and adequately decontaminated before reuse The inanimate environment such as floors and other surfaces may be heavily contaminated and acquisition of infection has been reported in a room that has been thoroughly cleaned. The excellent survival on drying and resistance to disinfectants increases the difficulty of removal of the organism on a surface. Although the role of the environment in transmission is uncertain, cleaning of heavily contaminated surfaces with a chlorine-releasing agent (1000 ppm av Cl) is usually recommended, as is thorough terminal cleaning.

General precautions include antibiotic restriction, especially of broad-spectrum agents, e.g. cephalosporins. Vancomycin should be used only for severe cases, since there is a risk of selecting resistant enterococci or possibly vancomycin-resistant MRSA.

Movement of patients from a potentially contaminated ward to other wards should be restricted. Rapid routine typing methods are not available, but 'fingerprinting' with mass spectrometry and molecular methods has been reported.

Infectious diseases of childhood (Madeley, 1995)

These commonly occur in paediatric wards and a succession of cases can occur in a ward over many months if adequate action is not taken. The common infections, chicken-pox, measles, rubella and mumps, can usually be readily identified and outbreaks are easily recognized by clinical means. The infected child should be isolated or sent home. If more than one, they can be nursed together in one ward. Susceptible children who may be harmed by the infection, e.g. leukaemics, those on steroids or other immuno-suppressive drugs or with chronic diseases of the chest, heart or kidneys, should be given gammaglobulin.

A particular problem is that of susceptible staff. If it is decided to keep the ward open to all admissions, an infected member of staff could be responsible for further cases, even if the original case was isolated before spread had occurred to other patients. It is preferable to employ staff who have had the disease, or have been immunized, e.g. against measles and rubella, but this is not always known. Female and male staff not immune to rubella should not work on paediatric, isolation or maternity wards. A major problem is in an isolation ward which includes infected and susceptible patients. Patients with chicken-pox or measles should not be nursed by staff who are also attending immunosuppressed patients unless there is reasonably certain evidence of previous infection or immunity.

Non-immune staff contacts of chicken-pox should preferably be excluded from maternity, paediatric, transplant and renal units from 10 to 21 days after exposure. Prophylaxis with acyclovir can also be considered for non-immune staff and they may be allowed to continue working, but possibly not in high-risk wards (Jones et al., 1997).

Respiratory syncytial virus spreads mainly by close contact. Handwashing between patients and wearing of gowns or aprons should reduce spread. Cohort nursing can be introduced if there are several cases, but is of doubtful value during a community outbreak in which new cases are continually being admitted. Spread to staff and back to a patient commonly occurs. In addition to handwashing, gloves for contact with secretions and wearing of an eye/nose protection reduce the risk of mucosal and conjuctival contamination and acquisition of infection by staff.

It is unnecessary to clean or disinfect wards after occupation by patients with childhood diseases as infection from the environment does not occur.

When to close wards is a difficult problem and is discussed on page 71.

Tuberculosis

It is usual to isolate patients with open pulmonary tuberculosis (i.e. with a positive ZN smear) for at least the first 2 weeks after commencing treatment (Department of Health, 1996). Isolation should be in a single room, preferably with extraction of air to the outside (e.g. with a window extraction fan or preferably with a ducted negative-pressure system of strains are multi-resistant). The period of isolation is uncertain, but from animal experiments and clinical experience the risk of spread after 2 weeks' effective treatment should be small and most of the organisms in the sputum should be non-viable. Exceptions will occur where the response is slow or the organisms are resistant to the antibiotics used, so that it is necessary to be careful in making hard and fast rules on length of time of isolation. A longer period of isolation (e.g. 4 weeks) should be carried out on paediatric wards or in patients with HIV infection.

Protecting the staff from acquiring respiratory infections by wearing masks is another uncertainty. It is unlikely that conventional masks will provide adequate protection, but may be advisable when dealing with severe disease. It may be more logical for the patient to wear the mask particularly when receiving close attention. Strains which are resistant to the common agents, especially to rifampicin and INAH, appear to be increasingly isolated in the USA, as well as in developing countries. Staff nursing these patients are recommended to wear good-fitting industrial-type masks with filters capable of removing small particles. The risks to staff immunized or naturally immune to tuberculosis appear to be small.

If a case of open pulmonary tuberculosis is found in a general ward, the immunity of the staff should be checked with the Occupational Health Department. Staff with a previously positive Mantoux or Heaf test or with evidence of successful BCG immunization require no further tests, but all contacts should be asked to report if they develop a chronic cough over the next 6 months. Staff who are tuberculin- or Heaf-test negative and have not received BCG vaccine should be chest X-rayed 6 weeks to 2 months after exposure. If the X-ray is negative, BCG should be given.

Patient contacts are more difficult as many may have gone home when the index case is identified. The general practitioners of known close contacts should be informed and patients told to visit them if symptoms occur. Spread from one patient to another is infrequent and following up large numbers of patients is of doubtful value as most have had limited or no close contact with the patient. However, the risk of spread is greater on paediatric wards, or from patients who are HIV positive, and follow-up of contacts is more important.

Other mycobacteria, e.g. *Myco. chelonae* or *Myco. avium intracellulare*, may cause respiratory or skin infections. These and other atypical mycobacteria are particularly likely to be isolated in HIV-infected and immunosuppressed patients. Spread can occur between patients, but often they are acquired from water supplies or bronchoscopes rinsed with contaminated water (see page 146).

Hepatitis B (HBV), hepatitis C (HCV) and human immuno-deficiency virus (HIV) infections

Although outbreaks of HBV are now rare in hospitals due to the introduction of immunization, screening of blood and blood products and improved prevention methods, the increased recognition of HCV and the continued presence of HIV requires routine preventive measures against bloodborne spread of these infections. However the risk of spread is low, provided that needle stick injuries are avoided and equipment is adequately decontaminated.

Since undetected carriers are likely to be admitted with another diagnosis, some universal precautions are necessary (see Chapter 7). These can vary with the risk and available equipment, but some should be adopted as routine procedures for staff. For example:

- Lesions on hands should be covered with a waterproof dressing.
- Gloves should be worn when carrying out invasive procedures, or if contact with blood or body fluids is likely. In hospitals where risks are low or in countries where gloves are in short supply, this recommendation may be modified, but handwashing is always necessary. This alone will considerably reduce the risk of acquiring or transmitting infection.
- If the skin or conjunctiva is contaminated with blood or any other body fluid, wash immediately and thoroughly.
- If splashing with blood is likely, e.g. during surgery, dentistry or delivery in obstetrics, goggles or safety spectacles and a plastic apron or other impermeable gown should be worn.
- Needles should be discarded immediately by the user into a puncture-proof container without recapping, unless a safe recapping or alternative technique is available.
- Sharp instruments should be handled with care during operations and not handed to the surgeon directly by the instrument nurse or vice versa.
- Blood spillage should be immediately cleaned and the operator should wear gloves. It may be preferred to disinfect the spillage, e.g. with a chlorine-releasing solution or powder containing 5000–10 000 ppm of av Cl, but rapid cleaning is of greater importance.

Other measures

- Blood and blood products should be screened for HBV, HCV and HIV.
- All staff carrying out invasive procedures or likely to be in contact with blood or body fluids, e.g. laboratory and post-mortem room staff, laundry and waste disposal staff as well as clinical staff, should be immunized against hepatitis B.

- Following an injury with a sharp instrument, bleeding should be encouraged from the site of injury, followed by thorough washing in running water. The supervisor should immediately be informed. If the instrument was used on a known HBV-positive patient, give hepatitis B immunoglobulin and a booster dose of vaccine if the antibody titre in the staff member is less than 10 units. Commence an immunization programme if the member of staff has not been immunized. If the instrument was used on a known HIV-positive patient, treatment with appropriate therapeutic agents, i.e zidovudine possibly combined with one or more other agents, should be commenced within 1–2 h and continued for 4 weeks. The advantages and disadvantages of continuation of therapy should be discussed with the member of staff as soon as possible after the first dose a 24 hour advisory system should be available.
- Staff carrying out exposure prone procedures should not be hepatitis e-antigen positive. The risk of transmission of infection from HB surface antigen, HCV or HIV staff carriers to patients by invasive procedures or other means is minimal. Health service staff should be able to continue to work normally, but impartial professional advice should be obtained both as a protection for the patient and the employing authority (UK Health Departments, 1998). However, little information on the transmission of HCV from staff is available.
- Single room isolation of patients with these bloodborne infections is unnecessary unless for other purposes, e.g. severe diarrhoea or pulmonary tuberculosis in AIDS patients. Most infections in AIDS patients, e.g. pneumocystis infection, are not hazardous to staff. HIV-positive women should be given zidovudine, possibly with another agent, before and after delivery. The newborn should be treated with oral drugs for 6 weeks. It has been claimed that this reduces the risk of infection in the newborn from 26% to 8%.

Transmissible spongiform encephalopathies – e.g. Creutzfeldt-Jakob disease, kuru, scrapie (sheep), BSE (mainly cattle)

Prevention of spread requires sterilization of surgical instruments by special procedures (see page 166) and care in handling tissues of the central nervous system, including formalin-fixed tissues. Spread by blood and other body fluids is unlikely, apart possibly from CSF, but routine blood precautions are usually advised and tissue donors are restricted. After skin contact with body fluids or tissues, wash well in water (Advisory Committee on Dangerous Pathogens, 1998).

Other infectious diseases

Potentially dangerous infectious diseases, such as diphtheria, are now rare in the UK, and a case tends to cause an excessive response in the staff unless everyone is informed of the risks. All departments likely to be involved such as the laundry, CSSD and domestic departments should be informed. Little action is required in the hospital other than prophylactic treatment of close contacts where appropriate, e.g. erythromycin for diphtheria, rifampicin or ciprofloxacin for meningococcal meningitis (not usually necessary for hospital staff). The CCDC should always be informed as investigations in families or schools may be necessary, and he/she has legal responsibilities for dealing with these infections.

Lassa fever, Ebola and other viral haemorrhagic diseases

Patients with these infections will usually be nursed in high-security infectious diseases units, but are likely to initially attend an accident or emergency unit or be admitted to a ward in a general hospital. A risk assessment is made of the suspected case, usually by an infectious diseases consultant, and categorized as high, moderate or minimal risk (Advisory Committee on Dangerous Pathogens, 1996). Patients assessed as minimal risk can be nursed with standard isolation procedures in a single room of a general hospital. Moderate risk patients should be admitted to an isolation hospital with intermediate facilities, or to a high-security unit, and high-risk patients should be admitted immediately to a high-security unit. A local policy should be agreed and an example is included below.

Infection spreads mainly by the blood and body secretions. Universal precautions should be sufficient, but in view of the high mortality the following measures are suggested:

Patient in an accident and emergency department

- The patient with the suspected infection should be transferred to a designated isolation room in the department and not allowed to leave until agreed by the Infection Control Doctor.
- The casualty officer or clinician diagnosing the infection should inform the duty consultant physician and the ICD who will inform an infectious diseases consultant if necessary and the CCDC.
- On instructions from the ICD, the senior nurse on duty will close the department to all further admissions and allow no patients or staff to leave if the risk is moderate or high. He/she will also inform the ICN, senior nursing officer on duty and the duty administrator.
- Before transferring to the isolation room, remove all unnecessary equipment except the box containing protective clothing from the room. A notice 'Strict isolation – do not enter' should be placed on the door. One person only should accompany the patient into the room (a doctor or nurse who has already had close contact with the patient). This person should dress in a long-sleeved disposable gown, cap, filter-type mask and overshoes. These articles are provided in a special box contained in the isolation room. Urine and faeces should be collected in a disposable pan or urinal and seal it in a plastic bag.

If the infectious diseases consultant thinks a diagnosis of viral haemorrhagic fever is likely he will arrange for the transfer of the patient to a special unit and inform the CCDC or public health medical officer on duty.
Then:

- The senior nurse, ICN and administrator will collect names and addresses of all contacts and allow them to leave on agreement with the CCDC. The ICN and Occupational Health Nurse will be responsible for tracing other hospital contacts and the CCDC for persons outside the hospital.
- After the patient is removed to the ambulance, the person attending the patient will remove protective clothing and seal it in a plastic bag, and leave the room. The door should be sealed until the CCDC has made arrangements for decontamination of the room and its contents and disposal of potentially infected materials, usually on advice from the ICT.
- The administrator will call a meeting of the Major Outbreaks Committee (CCDC, ICD and ICN, consultant physician, senior nurse and Occupational Health Nurse or Physician, see page 51).

Patient in a ward

- The doctor in charge will inform the consultant physician and the ICD, who will inform an infectious diseases consultant if necessary, and the CCDC.
- Transfer the patient to a side room.
- The senior nurse in the ward will inform the ICN (who will bring the box containing protective clothing) and the senior nursing officer on duty in the hospital.
- A notice 'Strict isolation – do not enter' is placed on the door. One doctor or nurse should accompany the patient into the ward and should dress in the protective clothing.
- Do not take any laboratory specimens until agreed by the infectious diseases consultant. It is likely, that tests will be required to exclude more common treatable infection, e.g. malaria and typhoid fever.

If the infectious diseases consultant thinks the suspected infection is likely he will arrange for transport to the special unit and inform the CCDC. The infection control and occupational health nurses will collect names of contacts, not forgetting laboratory staff who may have handled specimens, as well as radiology or physiotherapy staff where relevant. The CCDC will instruct the ambulance service on transport and decontamination requirements. The Major Outbreaks Committee will be called and decontamination procedures decided, as well as any quarantine arrangements.

The admission of a suspected patient to a general hospital should be avoided if possible. General practitioners should request a visit by the infectious diseases consultant to the patient's home.

Closure of wards

This is a major step which reduces the efficiency of the hospital and should rarely be necessary. Before making a decision to close a ward, it should be discussed by the outbreak group and a consensus obtained. A balance is required between the necessity of the clinical service to continue, e.g. intensive care, and the potential hazard of the infection to other patients, e.g. a virulent MRSA strain.

It should be unnecessary to close a ward for most staphylococcal or Gram-negative bacillary outbreaks, since single room isolation, good techniques and special control measures should prevent spread. If there are several cases and spread appears to be continuing, cohort nursing in a separate ward should be considered. However, recently there have been problems in controlling the spread of epidemic MRSA with measures that previously were effective. Consideration should be given to closure if existing procedures are failing to control spread and there is a significant risk to patients, e.g. in an orthopaedic ward, or if facilities for isolation nursing are inadequate, or numbers of nursing staff are insufficient, e.g. due to influenza.

To reduce the need for closure of an acute ward, every hospital should have adequate isolation facilities and preferably an isolation ward of at least 10 beds, particularly for children, cases of open pulmonary tuberculosis and epidemic MRSA. If the MRSA outbreak is large, a temporary isolation ward may be cost-effective.

Outbreaks of infectious diseases in paediatric wards present one of the major indications for ward closure. Should a ward be closed if a single case of chicken-pox is identified? Spread may not occur, but on the other hand an epidemic may continue for months, involving staff as well as children. An alternative may be to send home contacts in the early stages of the incubation period and to isolate long-stay non-immune contacts in an isolation ward, preferably with extract ventilation, between the 10th and 21st days after exposure. The ward could then remain open. This is particularly advantageous if it is a surgical ward.

Non-immune staff contacts should be similarly excluded from duty. Staff immunization will reduce this problem, e.g. for measles, but the chicken-pox vaccine, although apparently effective, is not yet routinely available in the UK. The prophylactic use of acyclovir may be considered (Jones *et al.*, 1997). However, if a disease is common in the community and cases are being continually admitted, e.g. RSV infections, closure may not be possible.

References and further reading

Advisory Committee on Dangerous Pathogens and Spongiform Encephalopathy Advisory Committee (1998) *Transmissible Spongiform Encephalopathy Agents.* Safe working conditions and the prevention of infection, London HMSO.

Advisory Committee on Dangerous Pathogens (1996) *Management and Control of Viral Haemorrhagic Fevers*, London, HMSO.

Anon (1977) *Drugs Therapeut. Bull.* Major advances in the treatment of HIV-1 infections. **35**, 25–29.

Ayliffe, G.A.J. (1996) *Recommendations for the Control of Methicillin-resistant Staphylococcus aureus (MRSA)*, Geneva, World Health Organisation. (WHO/EMC/LTS/96.1).

Ayliffe, G.A.J. (1997) The progressive intercontinental spread of methicillin-resistant *Staphylococcus aureus. Clin. Infect. Dis.*, **24** (suppl 1). S74–79.

Ayliffe, G.A.J., Lowbury, E.J.L., Geddes, A.M. and Williams, J.D. (1992) *Control of Hospital Infection: A Practical Handbook*, 3rd edn, London, Chapman and Hall.

Benenson, A.S. (1995) *Control of Communicable Diseases in Man*, 16th edn, New York, American Public Health Association.

Bloom, B.R. (1994) *Tuberculosis, Pathogenesis, Protection and Control*, Washington, ASM Press.

Cartmill, T.D.I., Panigrahi, H., Worsley, M.A. *et al.* (1994) Management and control of a large outbreak of diarrhoea due to *Clostridium difficile*. *J. Hosp. Infect.*, **27**, 1–15.

Casewell M.W. (1995) New threats to the control of methicillin-resistant *Staphylococcus aureus.* *J. Hosp. Infect.*, **30** (suppl.) 465–471.

Cox, R.A., Conquest, C., Mallaghan, C. and Marples, R.P. (1995) Major outbreak of methicillin-resistant *Staphylococcus aureus* caused by a new phage type (EMRSA 16). *J. Hosp. Infect.*, **29**, 87–106.

Damani, N.M. (1997) *Manual of Infection Control Procedures*, London, Greenwich Medical Media Ltd.

Department of Health (1995) *Hospital Infection Control: guidance in the control of infection in hospitals*, London, Department of Health.

Department of Health/Public Health Laboratory Service Working Group (1994) *The Prevention and Management of Clostridium difficile Infection* (PL(94) CO/4), London, Department of Health.

Department of Health (1996) *Recommendations for the Prevention and Control of Tuberculosis at Local Level*, The Interdepartmental Working Group on Tuberculosis. London, Department of Health.

Doebeling, B.N. (1993). Epidemics: identification and management. In *Prevention and Control of Nosocomial Infections* (R.P. Wenzex, ed.), Baltimore, Williams and Wilkins.

Fallon, R.J. (1994) How to prevent an outbreak of Legionnaires' disease. *J. Hosp. Infect.*, **27**, 247–256.

Health and Safety Executive (1995) *The Prevention and Control of Legionellosis*, Sudbury, Suffolk, HSE Books.

Jeffries, D.J. (1995) Viral hazards to and from health care workers. *J. Hosp. Infect.*, **30** (suppl.), 140–155.

Jones, E.M., Barnet, J., Perry, C. *et al.* (1997) Control of varicella-zoster infection on renal and other specialist units. *J. Hosp. Infect.*, **36**, 133–140.

Lowbury, E.J.L., Thom, B.T., Lilly, H.A. *et al.* (1970) Sources of infection with *Pseudomonas aeruginosa* in patients with tracheostomy. *J. Med. Microbiol.*, **3**, 39–56.

Madeley, C.R. (1995) Viral infections in children's wards – how well do we manage them? *J. Hosp Infect.*, **30** (suppl.), 163–171.

Mayhall, C. G. (ed.) (1996) *Hospital Epidemiology and Infection Control*, Baltimore, Williams and Wilkins.

Report of a Combined Working Party of the Hospital Infection Society and the British Society of Antimicrobial Chemotherapy (1998) Revised guidelines for the control of methicillin-resistant *Staphylococcus aureus* infection in hospitals. *J. Hosp. Infect.*, **39**, 253–290.

Report of a Combined Working Party of the British Society for Antimicrobial Chemotherapy and the Hospital Infection Society (1995). Guidelines on the control of methicillin-resistant *Staphylococcus aureus* in the community. *J. Hosp. Infect.*, **31**, 1–12.

Rhame, F.S. (1991) Prevention of nosocomial aspergillosis. *J. Hosp. Infect.*, **18** (suppl. A), 466–472.

Spicer, W.J. (1984) Three strategies in the control of staphylococci, including methicillin-resistant *Staphylococcus aureus*. *J. Hosp. Infect.*, **5** (suppl. A), 45–49.

UK Health Departments (1998) *Guidance from Clinical Health Care Workers: protection against infection with blood-borne viruses*, London, Department of Health.

Wade, J.J. (1995) The emergence of *Enterococcus faecium* resistant to glycopeptides and other standard agents – a preliminary report. *J. Hosp. Infect.*, **30** (suppl.), 483–493.

Wenzel, R.P., Nettleman, M.D., Jones, R.N. and Pfaller, M.A. (1991) Methicillin-resistant *Staphylococcus aureus*: implications for 1990s and effective control measures. *Am. J. Med.*, **91** (suppl. 3B) 221S–227S.

Wilson, P. and Dunn, L.J. (1996). Using an MRSA isolation scoring system to decide whether patients should be nursed in isolation. *Hyg. Med.*, **21**, 465–467.

5

Factors associated with surgical wound, chest, urinary tract, intravenous line infection and general measures for prevention

Surgical wounds

Infection may be acquired during the operation or postoperatively in the ward (see also Chapters 3 and 4). During the operation it may be acquired from the skin, respiratory or gastrointestinal tract of the patient, or from the skin or upper respiratory tract of the operating room staff, either by contact or through the air. Infection may also be acquired from contaminated equipment. Airborne spread is likely to be due to *Staph. aureus*, or possibly *Staph. epidermidis* in implant surgery (Lidwell *et al.*, 1983). Small numbers of *Staph. aureus* are usually present in the air of a normally ventilated theatre. The numbers falling into a wound during an operation are likely to be small, but a single skin scale may be carrying up to 100 or more individual cocci.

Factors influencing infection (Cruse and Foord, 1980)

The chances of a large enough inoculum reaching the wound and causing an infection are increased by the following:

- A long incision and a long operating time, as in cardiothoracic surgery.
- A heavy disperser of *Staph. aureus* in the theatre, especially if a member of the operating team.
- Many people in the theatre or considerable activity during the operation.
- The technique of the surgeon is inadequate and the wound edges are too tightly or loosely opposed; this may be difficult to avoid in obese patients. A haematoma may occur in the wound.
- The organisms land on an ischaemic area or an artificial implant.
- The wound is contaminated by the normal intestinal flora, e.g. during a colectomy.
- The wound is drained, particularly if drainage is not closed.
- The patient is particularly susceptible, e.g. very young, old, or has a pre-existing disease – cardiac, respiratory, diabetes, a malignant growth, or is suffering from malnutrition, obesity or is immunosuppressed.

Table 5.1   Risk assessment of acquisition of a wound infection in two patients*

Risk factors	Patient 1	Patient 2
Age	20	60
Sex	Female	Male
Wound infection	Clean undrained	Contaminated, drained
Preoperative stay in hospital	1 day	90 days
Special risks, e.g. diabetes	Nil	Yes
Risk of infection	0.3%	33.5%

* From Bibby et al. (1986) J. Hosp. Infect., 8, 31–39.

- The skin of the patient is colonized with a potential pathogen or there is an area of superficial sepsis on another site of the body.
- Preoperative shaving with a non-electric razor on the day before operation.

The hands of the surgeon or skin of the operation site are rarely colonized with *Staph. aureus*, and Gram-negative bacilli are usually removed by simple washing processes. The importance of glove punctures is over-emphasized in general surgery.

Although the host defences and surgical technique are the main factors, it must be ensured that:

1. The hands of the surgeon and the skin of the operation site are disinfected and no one with superficial sepsis is in the theatre.
2. The ventilation system is working efficiently (see page 197).
3. Instruments, operation gowns, drapes, etc. are sterile (rarely a problem).

Good surveillance will detect outbreaks and enable dispersers to be detected on subsequent investigation, and feedback of surveillance results to the surgeon can reduce infection, presumably by encouraging improvement in technique.

Short-term antibiotic prophylaxis is of value in contaminated or high-risk surgery, e.g. cardiac and joint prostheses, and operations should be individually assessed. Antibiotic prophylaxis should be given immediately before the operation, so that maximum antibiotic levels are present in the tissues during the operation.

The development of mathematical models based on multiregression analysis of risk factors which significantly influence the development of infection may enable the likelihood of infection to be predicted (Bibby et al., 1986; Table 5.1). These need further development since some of the data on factors are not available preoperatively or cannot be modified. Other models have been proposed (e.g. Culver et al., 1991), but all need a considerable amount of data to obtain a universally applicable model.

Ward-acquired infection

The place of acquisition of infection (i.e. ward or theatre) varies with different sites of operation and in different wards or hospitals. Clean and undrained wounds seal rapidly in 1–2 days and are unlikely to be infected in the ward.

It would seem that most infections are acquired in the operating theatre, but several ward factors are possibly relevant.

There is evidence of increasing ward infection rates with increased length of preoperative stay, with shaving on the day before operation or earlier and in drained wounds. The reason for the increased infection rate with increasing preoperative hospital stay is unknown. Originally it was considered to be due to the acquisition of more virulent hospital organisms, but this is probably unusual. Existing disease, requiring investigation and preoperative treatment, is a more probable explanation. Shaving on the day before operation may be responsible for colonization of small cuts, increasing the risks of wound infection. Shaving immediately before operation would not allow sufficient time for organisms contaminating the cuts to grow.

Preoperative bathing with an antiseptic is unlikely to prevent wound infection, since thorough disinfection of the operation site with an alcoholic solution at the time of operation will reduce more effectively the numbers of organisms on the skin. However, controlled studies with patients taking two or more baths or showers with chlorhexidine detergent have shown conflicting results (Lowbury, 1992).

In the presence of a staphylococcal outbreak, ward-acquired infections may be associated with overcrowding and staff shortages.

It seems rational to consider the following measures whenever possible:

1. Admit the patient to hospital as close to the time of operation as possible.
2. Shaving is usually unnecessary but excessive hair may be removed by clipping or depilation. If shaving is carried out, it should be done on the day of operation (Leaper, 1995).
3. Do not take ward bedding into the theatre.

    After operation:
4. Seal the wound for 1–2 days.
5. Use closed drainage system (if a drain is required).
6. Discharge the patient from hospital as soon as possible.

The likelihood of a wound becoming infected during a dressing change is slight, particularly if the wound is closed. However, there is some evidence that infections of high-risk wounds (e.g. cardiovascular) can occur in the recovery room and high aseptic standards are required.

Dressings should not be required on the wound after 48 h. If removed at this time or before, the conflict between nursing staff requiring good aseptic techniques and surgeons lifting dressings with their hands will not occur. A simplified technique for changing dressings could be developed (see Chapter 6). However, patients with wounds infected or colonized with potentially epidemic strains of *Staph. aureus* should be isolated in single rooms.

Lower respiratory tract infection

Hospital-acquired or associated respiratory tract infection may be endogenous or exogenous in origin. Postoperative infections are usually endogenous in patients with existing respiratory disease and are commonly caused by *Haemophilus influenzae* or *Strep. pneumoniae*. Instrumentation, e.g. by use of endotracheal or tracheostomy tubes, is an important risk factor for both endogenous and exogenous infection in which the normal respiratory defence mechanisms are bypassed (La Force, 1992). The organisms commonly associated with instrumentation or mechanical ventilation are Gram-negative bacilli, e.g. *Klebsiella* or *Enterobacter* spp., *Ps. aeruginosa, Serratia marcescens* and *Acinetobacter* spp., or Gram-positive cocci, e.g. *Staph. aureus*, especially MRSA. These organisms may be acquired from other infected or colonized patients on the hands of staff, less frequently from aerosols, or from food or from contaminated equipment.

Other risk factors (Chernet *et al.*, 1993; McGowan, 1996) include:

- severity of underlying illness
- old age
- coma
- surgical operations, especially of chest or abdomen
- major injuries
- obesity
- excessive smoking.

Infection is usually preceded by colonization of the oropharynx by antibiotic-resistant Gram-negative bacilli selected from the patient's own flora by antibiotic therapy, or from cross-infection.

The stomach may be colonized by Gram-negative bacilli, particularly in the absence of gastric acid due to H_2 blocking agents. Subsequent colonization of the oropharynx from gastric aspiration may occur. Aspiration of contaminated secretions from the oropharynx or stomach into the lung may then cause an infection. However, colonization in itself does not harm the patient and chemotherapy is only required for clinical infection. In addition, a biofilm may form on the surfaces of the endotracheal tube and organisms released from this may cause an infection. Clinical infection is often difficult to diagnose and is indicated by purulent sputum, pyrexia and radiological changes. Final diagnosis requires the isolation of the causative organism from transtracheal or bronchial aspirates or from protected brush cultures.

Endogenous infection is not readily prevented by the usual cross-infection measures, but may be prevented to some extent by physiotherapy. Avoiding the use of antibiotics will reduce the risk of selection of resistant organisms. A more controversial role for antibiotics is selective decontamination (SDD) of the oropharynx and stomach. Topical preparations, such as polymyxin, tobramycin and amphotericin B, are applied to the oropharynx and a systemic antibiotic, such as a cephalosporin, is usually also given parentally (Van Saene *et al.*, 1991). It is argued that as most infections are of endogenous origin and not prevented by the usual control of infection precautions, antibiotic prophylaxis is justified. The results have been variable, mortality is usually not reduced but the technique is frequently used with some success, particularly in trauma patients. The use of continuing broad-spectrum antibiotic prophylaxis is against all agreed principles for prevention of emergence of resistant strains and there is a considerable risk of highly resistant organisms emerging in an intensive care unit and creating major therapy and cross-infection problems. This risk can be reduced to some extent by efficient control of infection measures.

The essentials of prevention of Gram-negative cross-infection are: effective handwashing or disinfection between patients and a good aseptic technique, including wearing of gloves and using a sterile or adequately decontaminated catheter, for carrying out each suction technique (Creamer and Smyth, 1996). Hand disinfection with an alcohol rub is particularly useful in a busy intensive care unit. A separate gown or apron should be worn when attending an infected patient. Equipment, e.g. ventilators and associated tubing (changed every 48–72 h), humidifiers, washing bowls, shaving brushes, food-mixers and other items likely to come into close contact with the patient should be adequately decontaminated. Ventilators may be protected from contamination by the use of filters, reducing the need for routine decontamination between patients (see Chapter 11).

In addition to respiratory precautions, stopping antibiotics and isolation of patients with resistant strains are important steps in controlling an outbreak (see Chapter 13).

Urinary tract infection (see also Chapter 6)

Although infection can occur via the bloodstream, the commonest route is along the urethra. Infection without instrumentation is commoner in the female owing to the short urethra. However, hospital-acquired urinary tract infection usually occurs after instrumentation (Falkiner, 1993). The organisms are usually of faecal origin and may be found on the perineum or in the anterior urethra. Coagulase-negative staphylococci or micrococci are normally found in the anterior urethra and are a common cause of infection immediately after catheterization. Early infections are usually endogenous, but cross-infection occurs later in patients with an indwelling catheter. The use of a closed-drainage system considerably reduces the incidence of urinary tract infection in patients with indwelling catheters (Table 5.2), but infection still frequently occurs after about 7 or more days.

Organisms may reach the bladder along the outside of the catheter or along the lumen, possibly in an air bubble. They may gain access to the closed drainage system if the catheter is disconnected from the system or from the tap used to empty the bag.

It is not possible to define the main route of infection. In late infection spread along the outside of the catheter is likely, but attempts to prevent this by applications of topical antibiotics or disinfectants to the catheter–meatal junction have not been successful since the urethra is often colonized.

Table 5.2 Urinary tract infections in females with indwelling catheters*	
Treatment	Infection rate during drainage
Open drainage	29/34 (85%)
Closed drainage	18/47 (38%)
Closed drainage (with anchored catheter)	5/29 (17%)
* From Gillespie et al. (1967) Br. Med. J., 3, 90–92.	

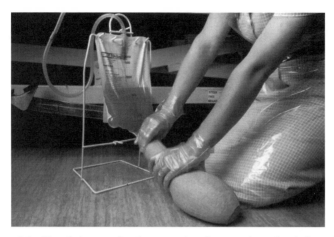

Figure 5.1 Use of gloves and a clean container for emptying urine drainage bag

Anchoring the catheter in females has achieved some success, as movement of the catheter in the short female urethra is a way of introducing infection. Retrograde spread from the bag or container along the lumen of the catheter is probably also important. Unfortunately, the non-return valve in the drainage bag is rarely effective. Tests in the laboratory in which a contaminated bag was tipped at intervals showed that growth reached the 'patient' end of the catheter in 2–3 days. Patients often sit on drainage bags. How do the organisms get into the bag? A few may be excreted in normal urine and grow in the drainage bag. Retrograde spread of large numbers of the patient's own organisms may cause a bladder infection. Although disinfectant in the bag may be considered useful, trials have not usually confirmed a preventative effect. Cross-infection from other patients is more important and is likely to occur via the hands of staff, contaminating the catheter–meatal junction, disconnecting the catheter, or contaminating the tap when emptying the drainage bag (Bradley *et al.*, 1986).

The fingers of the nurse are often contaminated with large numbers of organisms when emptying the bag and handling the container in which the bag is emptied (Figure 5.1). Unless the hands are thoroughly washed (or gloves are worn) between patients and a clean container is used, organisms are readily transferred to the next patient. The catheter–meatal junction may be contaminated when the patients use a toilet, commode or bedpan or during bathing. The hands of patients with a urinary infection are often heavily contaminated and may transfer infection to the hands of others who may subsequently contaminate their own catheter–meatal junction or perineum. Some organisms seem likely to spread, e.g. antibiotic-resistant *Klebsiella*. Cross-infection tends to occur if antibiotics are widely used in a unit and there are a number of patients with indwelling catheters, particularly if they are in adjacent beds or sit together during the day.

Infection may be acquired in non-catheterized patients, although the route of spread is uncertain. Contamination of urine bottles, bedpans and urine-testing equipment have all been associated with outbreaks. Contamination of tanks of disinfectant with Gram-negative bacilli have been reported on occasions.

It has been suggested that intermittent catheterization is less likely to be followed by infection than indwelling catheterization, but the evidence is limited. However, there is some evidence that infection after suprapubic catheterization is less than with an indwelling catheter.

General measures

Avoid catheterization if possible, particularly in incontinent patients. Remove the catheter as soon as possible (within 5 days). Collect urine specimens through an integral sampling point in the drainage set. Disinfect urinals and bedpans preferably by heat especially in urology wards, and wash hands between emptying bags (disinfection of hands with 70% alcohol is rapid and effective). It is also preferable to wear gloves. Containers in which drainage bags are emptied should be clean and dry (preferably disinfected by heat or disposable). Restriction in the use of broad-spectrum antibiotics (antibiotics are relatively ineffective in the presence of an indwelling catheter) is desirable, but a short prophylactic course to cover the instrumentation period may prevent bacteraemia and reduce infection in the first few days of continuous catheterization, particularly if the patient already has a urinary tract infection. In addition to the above measures, separation of patients with indwelling catheters in the ward is advisable during an outbreak. Isolate patients with highly resistant strains (Fryklund *et al.*, 1997). Introduce alcoholic disinfection of hands after handling infected patients or their immediate environment.

Infection of intravenous catheter sites

Infection may be local at the insertion site, e.g. thrombophlebitis, or systemic (septicaemia). Infections may be due to contamination of the infusion fluid or may arise during insertion of the cannula, or during maintenance of the administration of the fluid and of the insertion site (Elliott *et al.*, 1994; Pearson, 1996).

The infusion fluid may be contaminated from inadequate sterilization and subsequent growth of the surviving organisms. These are usually Gram-negative bacilli, such as *Enterobacter* spp., pseudomonads, *Citrobacter* spp. and *Serratia marcescens*. Occasionally other organisms, such as *Candida* spp., may grow in nutrient fluids used for parenteral nutrition. Staphylococci do not grow well in most intravenous fluids (see page 21). Contamination may also occur during addition of medicaments to the infusion fluid, but growth of contaminants usually does not take place unless the bag is left at room temperature for long periods (e.g. 12 h or longer). Infections of the insertion site are the most common and are usually caused by the patient's own skin organisms, e.g. *Staph. epidermidis* and less frequently by *Staph. aureus*. These skin organisms tend to colonize the outer and sometimes the inner surface of the cannula and are protected by a biofilm. Similar organisms may be introduced on the hands of staff when changing administration sets, injecting drugs into the tubing or injection port, or handling the cannula or insertion site. Occasionally transient hand contaminants, e.g. Gram-negative bacilli may be introduced by this route. The colonized cannula, or infected insertion site, may be associated with septicaemia or endocarditis in a susceptible patient.

Main risk factors for acquiring infection

- The length of time of catheterization.
- An inadequate aseptic technique (during insertion and subsequent maintenance).
- Triple lumen catheters.
- Parenteral nutrition.

Essential methods for prevention of infection

- Catheterization should be avoided whenever possible and should be used only on good clinical indications.
- Daily inspection of insertion site and removal of catheter if any signs of infection or for peripheral catheters at 72 h if a suitable alternative site is available. Always remove the catheter as soon as clinically possible.
- Handwashing or disinfection of hands of operator when inserting the catheter. Preferably apply 70% ethanol or isopropanol, with or without chlorhexidine or povidone-iodine, for at least 30 s, to the hands and rub to dryness.
- Thorough disinfection of skin of insertion site with 70% ethanol or isopropanol, with or without chlorhexidine or povidone-iodine before inserting the cannula. Apply for at least 1 min and allow to dry.
- Cover insertion site with dressing, preferably a clear semi-permeable dressing to allow easy inspection. Semi-permeable dressings should be changed at least every 3 days irrespective of the appearance of the site. This reduces the likelihood of growth of the resident flora in the possibly moist conditions under the dressing.
- Handwashing or disinfection before changing fluid container, or administration set or changing dressing.
- Secure device to skin to avoid movement of cannula. Experience and skill in inserting the cannula and maintenance of the infusion are of major importance. An intravenous team for the hospital will keep infections to a minimum, but if full time can be expensive.

References and further reading

Ayliffe, G.A.J., Lowbury, E.J.L., Geddes, A.M. and Williams, J.D. (1992) *Control of Hospital Infection: A Practical Handbook*, London, Chapman and Hall.

Bibby, B.A., Collins, B.J. and Ayliffe, G.A.J. (1986) A mathematical model for assessing risk of postoperative wound infection. *J. Hosp. Infect.*, **8**, 31–39.

Bradley, C.R., Babb J.R., Davies, J. *et al.* (1986) Taking precautions. *Nursing Times*, **82**, (suppl).

Chevret, S., Hemmer, M., Carlet, J., Langer, M. and the European Cooperative Group on Nosocomial Pneumonia (1993) Incidence and risk factors of pneumonia acquired in intensive care units. Results from a multicenter prospective study on 996 patients. *Intens. Care Med.*, **19**, 256–264.

Craven, D.E., Stega K.A. and La Force, F.M. (1988) Pneumonia. In *Hospital Infections* (J.V. Bennett and P.S. Brachman, eds), pp. 487–513, Philadelphia, Lippincott-Raven.

Creamer, E. and Smyth, E.G. (1996). Suction apparatus and the suctioning procedure: reducing the infection risks. *J. Hosp. Infect.*, **34**, 1–9.

Cruse, P.J.E. and Foord, R. (1980) The epidemiology of wound infection. A 10 year prospective study of 62,939 wounds. *Surg. Clin. N. Am.*, **60**, 27–40.

Culver, D.H., Horan, T.C., Gaynes, R.P. *et al.* (1991) Surgical wound infection rates by wound class, operative procedure, and patient risk index. *Am. J. Med.*, **91** (suppl. 3B), 152S–157S.

Elliott, T.S.J., Faroqui, M.H., Armstrong, R.F. and Hanson, G.C. (1994) Guidelines for good practice in central venous catheterization. *J. Hosp. Infect.*, **28**, 163–176.

Falkiner, F.R. (1993) The insertion and management of indwelling catheters – minimizing the risk of infection. *J. Hosp. Infect.*, **25**, 79–90.

Fryklund, B., Haeggman, S. and Burman, L.G. (1997) Transmission of urinary bacterial strains between patients with indwelling catheters – nursing in the same room and in separate rooms compared. *J. Hosp. Infect.*, **36**, 147–153.

Gillespie, W.A., Lennon, G.G., Linton, K.B. and Phippen, G.A. (1967) Prevention of urinary tract infection by means of closed drainage into a sterile plastic bag. *Br. Med. J.*, **3**, 90–92.

Leaper, D.J. (1995) Risk factors for surgical infection. *J. Hosp. Infect.*, **30** (suppl.), 127–139.

Lidwell, O.M., Lowbury, E.J.L., Whyte, W. *et al.* (1983) Bacteria isolated from deep joint sepsis after operation for total hip or knee replacement and the sources of infection with *Staphylococcus aureus. J. Hosp. Infect.*, **4**, 19–29.

Lowbury, E.J.L. (1992) Special problems in hospital antisepsis. In *Principles and Practice of Disinfection, Preservation and Sterilization* (A.D. Russell, W.B. Hugo and G.A.J. Ayliffe, eds), Oxford, Blackwell Scientific Publications.

Mayhall, C. G. (ed.) (1996) *Hospital Epidemiology and Infection Control*, Baltimore, Williams and Wilkins.

McGowan, J.E. (1996) Risk factors and nosocomial infection control. In *Surveillance of Nosocomial Infections* (A.M. Emmerson and G.A.J. Ayliffe, eds), Bailliere's Clinic Infect. Dis. Vol. 3, 159–306.

Pearson, M.L. (1996) Guidelines for the prevention of intravascular device-related infections. *Infect. Cont. Hosp. Epidemiol.*, **17**, 438–473.

Taylor, E.W. (ed.) (1992) *Infection in Surgical Patients*, Oxford, Oxford University Press.

Van Saene, H.K.F., Stoutenbeek, C.P. and Hart, C.A. (1991) Selective decontamination of the digestive tract (SDD) in intensive-care patients: a critical evaluation of the clinical, bacteriological and epidemiological benefits. *J. Hosp. Infect.*, **18**, 261–267.

Ward, V., Wilson, J., Taylor, L. *et al.* (1997) *Preventing Hospital-acquired Infection. Clinical Guidelines*, London, Public Health Laboratory Service.

Wilson, A.P.R., Weavill, C., Burridge, J. and Kelsey, M.C. (1990) The use of the wound scoring method 'ASEPSIS' in postoperative wound surveillance. *J. Hosp. Infect.*, **16**, 297–309.

6

Nursing aspects of prevention of infection: aseptic and hygienic techniques

Relating infection control to nursing practice

Infection control practices need to be integrated into the nursing procedures of each hospital. This means that problems of infection control should be identified in each clinical area and included in the care plans for individual patients. The equipment and procedures used will vary from one hospital to another and will need to be critically assessed to ensure that infection risk has been minimized. Methods should be sufficiently flexible to adapt to patient needs without increasing that risk. Although infections are classified as wound, urinary tract, enteric infections, etc., it is important to remember that it is an individual who becomes infected and that the infection is likely to cause emotional as well as physical distress. Unnecessary measures can exaggerate the severity of the problem in the minds of the patients, their families and friends. Wherever practical, the reason for the measures taken should be explained in a language appropriate to the individual. Measures applied to an infected patient are often taken to protect other more vulnerable patients, and the risk to families and visitors may be very low. Explaining this can be reassuring to the infected patient and relatives.

Each patient should be seen as part of the nursing environment interacting in a specific way with that environment and the other patients. The presence of a patient may increase infection risk to others, or other patients may increase the risk to him/her. The distribution of patients within the ward can be important even where isolation is not required.

The complexity of this interaction is apparent when considering individual patients. An elderly lady recovering from a hip prosthesis operation is likely to be vulnerable to a different range of organisms from those infecting a patient following colonic surgery. Her age may make her more vulnerable than a much younger person having the same operation. She may be particularly vulnerable to developing pressure sores. Should this happen, the pressure sores are likely to be colonized by potential pathogens and, apart from the risk to herself, she becomes a potential source of infection to other patients. Previous antibiotic treatment for chronic bronchitis may have caused colonization of carriage sites with antibiotic-resistant organisms which could increase infection risk both to the patient and others in contact with her. Catheterization may become necessary. About one-third of all hospital-acquired infections are of the urinary tract, most of which are associated with catheterization. Nursing care must be planned with an awareness of the measures that increase infection risk, and the use of these techniques balanced against the possible benefits. The care plan for this patient could include a high fluid intake and frequent opportunities to empty her bladder, so that catheterization can be avoided; frequent mouth toilet to prevent oral thrush; frequent turning, attention to pressure areas and the use of pressure-relieving devices to prevent bed sores; early mobilization to prevent chest infection. Infection control measures need to be related to the requirements of each individual patient. Appropriate measures will not be the same for each patient, and even when the same measure is adopted for several patients, the priority given to that measure may be different. It is a waste of valuable resources to apply unnecessary infection control measures, but failure to apply necessary ones may indicate a lack of professional judgement.

Risk assessment

It should therefore be part of the nursing process to assess the infection risk for each individual patient. It is too easy to neglect infection among the many other priorities. A decision that 'it is not really necessary to wash the hands on this occasion' or 'the drainage tap on the urine bag has touched the floor, but I haven't got time to change it now. It will probably be all right' or 'he's complaining of pain at the site, but the dressing isn't due to be changed yet. I'll do it later' is often made. Such decisions on priorities are required, but it is important to be aware that decisions on acceptable risks are being made on the patients' behalf and not for the convenience of staff; the patient, not the nurse, becomes infected if the decision is wrong.

A hazard is something with the potential to do harm; risk is a measure of the probability of that happening. Health care is a risk activity. The decision to take a risk should be a positive one, based on good information on the possible consequences, and with the knowledge and consent of the patient. A decision not to wash hands due to pressure of work when they should be washed is a risky decision with which the patient might not agree. Patients carry with them to a greater or lesser extent an inherent risk or vulnerability to infection. In making a risk assessment the immunological competence of the patient, the medical condition, the procedures which can reasonably be expected to be carried out during the hospital stay, need to be taken into consideration. The environment in which those procedures will be carried out and other individuals who will share the environment with the patient are also relevant to risk.

Most hospital infections occur because the patient was exposed to micro-organisms when particularly vulnerable. The organisms involved are rarely unusual in virulence or other properties, but are able to reach a normally inaccessible susceptible site on the patient because of a particular procedure. Approximately 60% of hospital-acquired infections are caused by common Gram-negative bacteria that are either normal inhabitants of the gut or can be found in almost any used or static fluid, i.e. opportunistic pathogens. Other more specific human infections, e.g. childhood infectious diseases, may be acquired in hospital because the chance of contact is increased, often at a time when the ability to resist infection is decreased. This decrease may be due to disease, e.g. leukaemia, HIV infection or to the use of drugs which reduce immunological competence. It is because infection risk is associated with the reaction of the individual to his environment that advice may sometimes appear inconsistent; apparently irrelevant questions may be asked by infection control specialists in an attempt to establish which set of interactions are relevant on any specific occasion.

Risks will also vary in relative importance, and priorities will depend on the number of people likely to be infected, the severity of the resulting infection and how readily the infection responds to treatment. A hospital chef with *Salmonella* infection could infect hundreds, if not thousands, of people if catering practice is poor. A single case of diphtheria may require immediate action since the consequence of spread could be severe. The nurse with an uncovered infected finger could cause infections in many of the wounds of patients who had been dressed by her over the next few days. Accidentally touching a sterile dressing during a dressing procedure could infect the patient, but the probability is not high. Transferring *Staph. aureus* to cutlery while handing it to a patient could infect him/her, but the probability is again so remote that it can usually be ignored. Resources devoted to preventing infection should be related to the degree of risk involved.

Infection control may not be the major factor to be considered when carrying out a procedure and, where action is required, the wider implications must also be considered. It is normally advised that the same nurse should not attend an infectious patient and a heavily immunosuppressed patient on the same shift. This instruction may, however, be justifiably overridden in a sufficiently severe medical emergency, e.g. a cardiac arrest. In such a circumstance it would be unwise to spend time washing the hands before taking action.

Seeking advice

The ICN should be a readily available source of advice, and it is a major part of her role to interpret policies; if in doubt – ask. Do not, however, be surprised if you are then asked questions; the question of which disinfectant to use may be inappropriate for a situation in which cleaning may be sufficient or sterilization may be necessary. Where recommendations are made to cope with new problems, feedback is essential. Did it work and is it likely to occur sufficiently often to include in procedure manuals or codes of practice?

Measures to prevent infection

Infection control procedures may be generalized guidelines or policy decisions which may be non-clinical, e.g. catering, domestic practice, laundering, waste disposal, etc., or clinical, e.g. policies for isolation of patients, use of antibiotics, etc., or involve both clinical and non-clinical areas, e.g. disinfection policies. There may also be detailed guidance for specific procedures, e.g. catheterization. Policies should be sufficiently comprehensive to cover most common eventualities, easily followed and unambiguous. They should also be well publicized and readily available. Some flexibility to allow policies to be adapted for the requirements of individual patient care is required. Nurses should make themselves aware of existing policies when changing from one ward to another or from one hospital to another.

Handwashing in wards

Handwashing or disinfection is the most important technique in the prevention of cross-infection (Casewell and Phillips, 1977). However, apart from the studies of Semmelweiss and one or two studies in neonatal nurseries, there is little statistical evidence from controlled trials to confirm this statement. Many investigations have demonstrated the control of an outbreak by improving handwashing techniques, but this has usually been in association with other measures. Nevertheless, it is rational to consider that the hands of staff represent one of the main routes of spread. The problems to be considered are agents and techniques used and indications for handwashing.

Laboratory studies have demonstrated that washing with soap and water will remove or kill approximately 99% (10^2), antiseptic detergents approximately 10^2–10^3 and 60–70% alcohol 10^3–10^4 of transient organisms from the hands (Table 6.1). Although statistically significant differences between washing with soap and a disinfectant may be obtained, the clinical relevance of a statistical difference log 0.5–1.0 is much less certain.

Interpretation of laboratory results is difficult and the results should be assessed as indications of the order of effectiveness rather than an indication of specific reductions of organisms likely to be obtained under practical circumstances. Determining a clinically significant difference between a soap and water wash and an antiseptic wash would require a very large and expensive controlled study, which would probably add very little to our existing knowledge. Following a contaminated procedure, e.g. cleaning up after an incontinent patient, bacterial counts of up to 10^7 may be isolated from washings from the hands of the attendant. The reductions obtainable even with alcohol may be inadequate and gloves should be worn for such procedures.

The average time of handwashing varies between 10 and 20 s and a thorough wash covering all surfaces is important. In a study of blindfolded

Table 6.1   Hygienic hand disinfection (*E.coli* applied to finger tips*)

Preparations	No. of tests	Mean log reduction
70% Isopropanol	9	3.3
70% Ethanol	5	2.7
4% Chlorhexidine detergent	2	2.9
7.5% Povidone-iodine	4	2.5
2% Triclosan detergent	2	2.3
Unmedicated soap	13	2.1

* From Ayliffe *et al.* (1988a) J. Hosp. Infect., 11, 226–243.

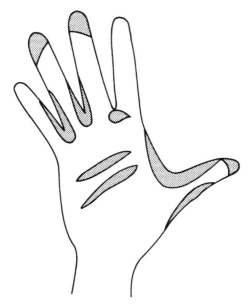

Figure 6.1   Areas commonly missed with poor handwashing technique (□). Demonstration of poor handwashing technique by use of dye.

nurses handwashing with a dye, certain areas were commonly missed (Taylor, 1978; Ayliffe *et al.*, 1978) (Figure 6.1). A suitable technique has been described to ensure adequate coverage of hands.

Nurses and other health care workers wash their hands much less frequently than expected and efforts are continually made to improve the frequency. However, it is not known whether this would influence the infection rate and too much washing will damage the skin.

Assessment of indications for handwashing will provide practical guidelines, although it is accepted some discrepancies will occur. A useful guide to deciding when a handwash is appropriate is to imagine that the next thing to be done is eat a sandwich. Studies in our laboratory using finger impressions have shown that significant hand contamination with patient strains is infrequent following contact with furniture, taking pulse, temperatures, bed-making, etc., but may occur following care of incontinent patients, emptying urine bags, bedpans, etc., or after bed-bathing or handling bedding from infected or colonized patients (Table 6.2).

Washing with soap and water should be sufficient for most procedures, but an antiseptic detergent may be preferred in special units or during outbreaks. Alcohol disinfection provides additional protection and can be introduced during outbreaks or where rapid disinfection is required, e.g. during rounds of patients, particularly when handwashing facilities are inadequate. The thoroughness of application is more important than the time spent on washing or the agent used.

Table 6.2   Pathogens on nurses' hands after ward procedures and after washing with chlorhexidine detergent

Procedure	Number of hands sampled	Number of hands showing			
		Staph. aureus		Gram-negative bacilli	
		Before washing	After washing	Before washing	After washing
Dressing change	11	5	1	0	0
Bed-making	10	1	0	0	0
Bed-bathing	15	6	1	1	1
Handling bedpans	29	12	1	4	1

Aseptic techniques

Many procedures are defined as aseptic techniques, e.g. catheterization, tracheal suction, wound dressings, etc. Usually this implies the use of sterile equipment, avoidance of direct contact with the susceptible site and other measures to reduce the probability of introducing potential pathogens into a susceptible site. Procedures may vary widely from one hospital to another though attempts to standardize them have been made (Ward *et al.*, 1997). Remaining differences may be due to financial restraint or personal preference, but procedures should be rational, each step should be justifiable and techniques should be kept up to date taking full account of any relevant research.

Wound dressings
The most commonly used aseptic technique is a wound dressing. Wounds can be divided into two main categories, surgical and traumatic. The main difference between these is that surgical wounds are usually produced under carefully controlled conditions intended to prevent the access of microbes and are then carefully closed under the same conditions. The traumatic wound may be heavily contaminated with organisms at the time of injury and may contain extraneous foreign matter and dead tissue likely to encourage subsequent infection. Burns are perhaps an exception for, though clearly traumatic, they are likely to be initially sterile but because of a large area of damaged skin readily become colonized.

Surgical sepsis is more likely to be acquired at the time of operation rather than in the ward, since it is more difficult for organisms to gain access to a closed wound. The organisms causing postoperative wound infection are more likely to be derived from the patient (autogenous) than from the operating team or the theatre environment (see Chapter 5). Drained wounds are more likely to become infected especially if an open drain is used, but there would appear to be little increase in infection risk if a closed drainage system is used. It is now rare for large, open or corrugated drains to be used. Infection rates are also likely to be high where there is leakage from the gut or other organs containing bacteria or where there is contact with another colonized or already infected site during the operation.

Open drains and heavily discharging wounds cause additional nursing problems. Prolonged wetting of the skin by exudate and frequent removal of dressings can damage the skin, reducing the rate of healing and increasing the likelihood of infection. As soon as exudate appears on the outer surface of the dressing it should be changed, as it will no longer prevent bacteria on the outer surface from reaching the wound, and if the wound is already infected, the moist exudate on the dressing surface will contaminate hands or other surfaces coming into contact with it. Many measures may be taken to prevent damage to the surrounding skin, but traditional remedies such as oatmeal paste, etc., may merely provide additional nutrition for bacterial growth. Many specialized commercial dressings are available but it would be expensive and impractical to carry stocks of each. A representative of each type should be chosen. However, these dressings should only be used when there is a relevant specific advantage in using that particular type of dressing for an individual patient. Bags similar to colostomy bags are sometimes used to contain copious exudate and do have some advantages but they do not entirely overcome the problem. They require frequent emptying and this may still lead to skin damage. Many trusts now have access to a clinical nurse specialist in tissue viability or wound care. Her advice should always be sought for complicated wounds.

Procedures may become out of date and require re-evaluation. It has long been recommended that all cleaning and bed-making should cease before wound dressings are carried out or intravenous catheters are inserted. This was intended to prevent airborne contamination of the exposed site. Although this is the preferred practice, these measures have become impractical. Changes in nursing practice mean that wound dressings are likely to be carried out at irregular intervals throughout the day and changes in domestic practice mean it is often not possible to delay cleaning procedures. Table 6.3 shows that even when substantial disturbance of bed linen occurs, the increase in airborne counts would be unlikely to greatly increase infection risk. In the same series of experiments, liquid culture medium was left exposed for short periods in a skin ward where large numbers of heavily contaminated skin scales are dispersed. The number of organisms recovered suggested that indirect transfer on to dressing trolley surfaces or instruments by the airborne route is unlikely to be a problem. Transfer on the hands of staff is likely to be much greater.

In non-touch techniques where forceps or gloves are used to avoid skin contact with the patient or the sterile dressings, the same effect can be obtained by using a gloved hand or by inverting a plastic bag over the dressing so that it is enclosed without direct contact with the hand. These

Table 6.3 Contamination from airborne organisms

Site sampled	Numbers of micro-organisms settling in 5 min, during			
	Bed-making	Shaking curtains	High activity	Wet cleaning
Cotton gauze (60 cm²)	19.8	8.4	27.0	2.4
Forceps (approx. 10 cm²)	3.3	1.4	4.5	0.4

methods are easier than manipulating forceps. There are perhaps many other techniques that could be re-evaluated. It is often taught that dressing techniques are carried out by two nurses, but experience suggests the second nurse is rarely available. This may leave the nurse to adapt the technique to a one-nurse dressing technique without proper knowledge of the most important infection control aspects. It would be preferable if nurses were taught a deeper understanding of the principles behind the techniques so that they could adapt them for a one-nurse technique safely when required. Nurses will often leave the bedside in the middle of a dressing to wash the hands, and the wound will be exposed for a longer period than is necessary. Handwashing may not be required at that time or alcohol could be applied at the bedside (Kelso, 1989).

The necessity of routine cleaning of wounds is doubtful. The exudate may have a useful antimicrobial effect and the cleaning procedure may only redistribute the organisms rather than remove them, irrespective of the method used (Thomlinson, 1987). Moreover, a cold cleansing solution lowers the temperature of the wound and disrupts wound healing. If cleaning is considered necessary, warm sterile saline is usually preferable to antiseptics as these, especially hypochlorites, e.g. Eusol may delay healing. The exposure time is also likely to be inadequate to obtain effective antibacterial action. Gloved or disinfected hands tend to be more effective than forceps for cleaning the wounds and it has been shown that little contamination of fingers occurs when using disinfected hands. Studies have previously demonstrated a significant reduction in infection when using a non-touch technique, but recent evidence shows that it can at least be modified.

As long as the package remains dry and intact the contents of dressing packs should remain sterile. They should be examined for evidence of damage or moisture penetration immediately before use, and if these are found, the pack should be returned to the Sterile Services Department. Other items on the dressing trolley are usually single use. The inner surface of a roll of adhesive tape is unlikely to present a major infection problem and it would usually be acceptable to use non-sterile adhesive tape on intact skin.

There are many functions of a dressing and it is necessary to understand why the dressing is being applied in a particular instance; if it is to protect while healing takes place, the amount of padding may be important; if it is to promote healing, then a gauze dressing that will remove the growing tissues along with the gauze is unsuitable. If the dressing is to protect against infection and prevent the organisms getting in or out, is it then sufficiently impermeable, or if the wound is discharging is it sufficiently absorbent to prevent strike through before the next dressing change? Where a patient requires surgery but has another infected site, occluding that site with transparent film dressing may prevent spread of the organism to the clean operation site and allow surgery to be carried out earlier than would otherwise be possible.

Not all wounds require aseptic techniques. There would seem little point in carrying out a rigorous aseptic technique on a colonized pressure sore, or even when dressing a surgical wound if the patient has just had a bath with the wound uncovered. The presence of dead tissue can prevent antibiotics or antiseptics reaching infecting organisms and can allow reduced oxygen tension which may allow anaerobes such as *Cl. perfringens* to multiply. The presence of slough will also delay healing, but care is necessary in the use of desloughing agents that may delay healing. The greater the understanding of the interaction between the wound surface, the microbe and the individual patient, the more likely it becomes that the right treatment will be selected.

Intravenous catheterization

The intravenous insertion site is a break in the natural defences through which fluids are introduced into the circulation via a needle or cannula. Organisms can enter the circulation from a contaminated fluid or giving set, or can grow along the outer or inner surface of the cannula (see page 81).

Bloodstream infections associated with intravenous lines are not uncommon. The incidence of infection can be minimized by careful attention to detail and sound aseptic practice. Many nurses are now trained to insert intravenous cannulae, thus providing continuity of care. Some trusts also have access to nurse specialists in intravenous therapy. Their expertise can be invaluable.

Contamination may also be introduced via injection ports. This potential hazard for introducing organisms remains controversial, but care is necessary to avoid the entry of organisms by this route. Containers of intravenous fluids are usually changed before significant growth occurs, but the giving set should be changed every 48–72 h.

The introduction of a cannula requires the same precautions as a surgical operation, e.g. thorough disinfection of the site and non-touch technique. This is particularly important for long-term catheterization. The hands should be disinfected with alcohol and sterile gloves should be worn. The skin of the insertion site should be disinfected with alcoholic chlorhexidine or another alcohol-based antiseptic. Bandages and dressings may create moist conditions suitable for bacterial growth and a clear adhesive bacteria-impermeable, water-vapour-permeable dressing may be preferred. This also allows observation of the site without removing the dressing. Movement of the cannula in the vein should be avoided by secure taping or use of dressings designed to meet this objective. However, some studies have shown an increase in bacterial growth under these dressings, but this may be reduced by reducing the skin flora to a low level before applying the dressing. The daily application of antiseptics or antibiotics to the insertion site has given variable results and the value remains doubtful.

Prevention of infection remains a problem and new approaches are required. A cannula surface to which organisms do not adhere, or the introduction of antimicrobial agents into the catheter material, are possibilities. However, avoiding cannulation or removal as soon as possible (or at least at 72 h) is the best method of preventing infection. Indications for cannulation need to be clearly identified, clinically justified and recorded in the clinical notes. It is equally important that removal of the cannula is recorded.

Urinary catheterization (see also page 78)

The insertion of a urinary catheter is usually done with care, since the infection risks are well understood. However, the benefits can be lost by poor management of the catheter and drainage bag. The flutter valve may prevent urine flowing from the bag to the tubing, but does not prevent urine in the tubing running back into the bladder. Generally, urimeters do not have flutter valves. The drainage bag should not be raised above bladder height without first clamping the tubing. Again, there are practical difficulties: bags may not be supplied with clamps; gate clips and Spencer Wells forceps may disappear. Not only nurses handle drainage bags: physiotherapists often pin bags above waist height when mobilizing the patient; domestic staff may rest the bag on the bed while cleaning the floor.

The collection of a catheter specimen of urine is simplified by incorporating a sample point in the tubing. Provided a small-bore needle is used, samples can be taken direct from latex catheters, since the material of the catheter and sample point are similar.

A technique which is on the borderline between hygienic and aseptic is emptying of urine drainage bags. This is a task commonly allocated to junior members of staff who may not be aware of the risk to the patient. Use of drainage bags with taps has helped to reduce the incidence of urinary tract infection associated with indwelling catheters. Frequent disconnection at the catheter–bag junction was thought to be a major source of contamination. However, the taps themselves present a hazard and illustrate the point that every action has an influence on the system as a whole. If the tap is allowed to drag on the floor or is contaminated by handling, micro-organisms can track back into the urine in the bag. This acts as a culture medium. The flutter valve does not necessarily prevent urine in the tubing becoming contaminated. If the bag is raised above bladder height, contaminated urine will run back into the bladder. The use of disinfectant (chlorhexidine or hydrogen peroxide) in the drainage bag should prevent the growth of organisms, but its use remains controversial.

It is usual to recommend regular meatal toilet at 4–8-hourly intervals for those with indwelling catheters. It is a time-consuming, and though a simple procedure is often seen as one that can be neglected if the ward is busy. Is frequent cleaning necessary? There is evidence to suggest that daily meatal toilet is adequate. Similar to emptying the bag, it is a procedure on the borderline between aseptic and hygienic. The catheter drains a 'sterile' body cavity and the equipment used is sterile, but the technique is hygienic. It is probably most conveniently done at the time of the daily bath, using pre-packed sterile equipment and freshly drawn tap water. This would not be necessary if the patient can use the ward bath or shower, and is an example of balancing the effort involved against the size of the risk. While there may be some risk in using the bath, it is probably less than the risk of not having a bath. Whether the risk can be reduced by adding an antiseptic solution to the water is uncertain.

It is surprising so many uncertainties remain in the prevention of infection in catheterized patients. Avoiding the use of a catheter and removal as rapidly as possible from catheterized patients, remain the most certain methods of preventing or reducing infection. The use of absorbent pads rather than a catheter has been shown to reduce infection as has suprapubic drainage.

Table 6.4   Viable Gram-negative bacteria isolated from stored wet and dry wash bowls filled for patient bed-baths

No. of organisms per ml	Number of bowls sampled	
	Wet	Dry
10^3	11 (22%)	47 (94%)
10^3–10^7	39 (78%)	3 (6%)
Total	50	50

Bathing the patient

Bathing is an important routine procedure for patient comfort and to reduce infection risk. However, it should be carried out with care. It is better to clean towards the naturally heavily contaminated areas such as the rectum so that Gram-negative bacteria are not distributed over the rest of the body surface, though they will not survive long on an intact, dry skin in good condition. It is always preferable to use a fresh disposable wipe and the same cloth should never be used on more than one patient. Unless a fresh, disposable wash cloth is used each time, the patient may be microbiologically dirtier at the end of the bath than at the beginning.

Gram-negative organisms die on drying. A dry skin is unlikely to be colonized by Gram-negative bacilli, but patients confined to bed tend to have moist, sweaty skin in the area under the bedclothes. If wash bowls are left clean but wet and stacked, they act as incubators and bacteria multiply in the moisture trapped between the layers of bowls (Table 6.4). Therefore, bowls are contaminated even before use. Contaminated wash bowls have been implicated in an outbreak of infection.

When wards are under pressure, it is common practice not to change the water during a bed-bath, and to use the same wash cloth for all areas of the body. By the end of the bath, the water is a soup of soap and bacteria. This presents a potential hazard if the patient has a break in the skin, e.g. surgical wound, wound drain, intravenous cannula.

Oral toilet

This is a frequent and necessary procedure, but not an aseptic one. It is an example of a hygienic measure, and is particularly important for patients with nasogastric tubes, the unconscious, the immunosuppressed and those on broad-spectrum antibiotics. It is a hygienic rather than an aseptic technique, since it does not significantly breach the body's defences, rather it enhances them. Oral *Candida* infections are a common complication of debilitated patients. Chest infections are sometimes associated with nasogastric tubes since they breach the barrier between the oesophagus and trachea. Patients regurgitate and aspirate small quantities of stomach contents. Cleaning the mouth also stimulates production of saliva, a mild antiseptic, and removes crust and debris in which organisms can multiply. Since the mouth is not a sterile area, equipment used can be clean rather than sterile. Gloves should be worn because some infectious agents may be present in the mouth or saliva, e.g. herpes, hepatitis B.

Summary

Though Florence Nightingale did not subscribe to the germ theory of infection, she did recognize the importance of sound hygiene. However, it is difficult to adopt the most sensible measures if the knowledge of hygiene is based on folklore and ritual. Nurses who choose infection control as their specialism soon learn to recognize that learning the scientific theory behind good practice can be easier than unlearning the ritual and abandoning the prejudices. The amount of practice that is based on sound theory and has been scientifically evaluated is increasing but much ritual and prejudice remains (Walsh and Ford, 1989). Some unnecessary practices have been abandoned and others are being re-evaluated. The wearing of caps, masks and gowns for routine dressings has been abandoned, as has the use of masks for deliveries and for use when handling premature babies; this has been done without increasing infection rates. The ritual cleaning of the trolley before every dressing is another wasteful procedure which has largely been abandoned.

References and furthers reading

Anon. (1991) Local applications to wounds–2. Dressings for wounds and burns. *Drug Therapent. Bull.*, **29,** 27.

Ayliffe, G.A.J., Babb, J.R., Davies, J. *et al.* (1988) Hand disinfection and comparison of various agents in laboratory and ward studies. *J. Hosp. Infect.*, **11,** 226–243.

Ayliffe, G.A.J., Babb, J.R. and Quoraishi, A.H. (1978) A test for hygienic hand disinfection. *J. Clin. Path.*, **31,** 923–928.

Bradley, C.R., Babb, J.R., Davies, J. *et al.* (1986) Taking precautions. *Nurs. Times*, **82** (suppl.), 70–73.

Casewell, M.W. and Phillips, I. (1977) Hands as a route of transmission of *Klebsiella* species. *Br. Med. J.*, **2,** 1315–1317.

Horton, R. and Parker, L. (1997) *Informed Infection Control Practice*, Edinburgh, Churchill Livingstone.

Infection Control Nurses Association (1997) *Information Resources*, 2nd edn, Harpenden, SDS Media Print.

Kelso H. (1989) Alternative technique. *Nurs. Times*, **85** (23), 68–72.

Meers, P., McPherson, M. and Sedgwick, J. (1997) *Infection Control in Healthcare*, 2nd edn, Cheltenham, UK, Stanley Thornes.

Taylor, L.J. (1978) Evaluation of handwashing techniques, parts 1 and 2. *Nurs. Times*, **74,** 54–56 and 108–110.

Thomlinson, D. (1987) To clean or not to clean. *J. Infect. Cont. Nurs.*, **35,** 71–75.

Ward, V., Wilson, J., Taylor, L.J. *et al.* (1997) *Preventing Hospital-acquired Infection. Clinical Guidelines*, London, PHLS.

Walsh, M. and Ford, P. (1989) *Nursing Rituals: Research and Rational Actions*, Oxford, Butterworth-Heinemann.

Wilson, J. (1995) *Infection Control in Clinical Practice*, London, Bailliere Tindall.

Worsley, M.A., Ward, K.A., Parker, L. *et al.* (eds) (1990) *Infection Control Guidelines for Nursing Care*, London, ICNA.

7

Nursing aspects of prevention of infection: isolation

Isolation precautions in context

Isolation, the separation of an infectious person from other people, is possibly the oldest form of infection control still practised. The veneer of rationality over modern practice is but a thin covering for a host of perceptions, values, beliefs and attitudes derived from the ignorant past rather than the evidence-based present. In the introduction to the US 'Guideline for isolation precautions in hospitals', the authors write: 'Because there have been few studies to test the efficacy of isolation precautions and gaps still exist in the knowledge of the epidemiology and modes of transmission of some diseases, disagreement with some of the recommendations is expected' (HICPAC, 1996). Writing in 1993, Garner and Hierholzer say: 'As such, isolation precautions continue in most cases to be based on theoretical rationale and perceptions of what is possible, practical, and prudent for all concerned.' Even earlier, Williams (1970) wrote: 'We could devise any number of elaborate preventive measures, but even if money were unlimited, the ability of hospital personnel to observe a plethora of precautions is limited. . . . It should be our aim . . . to determine those procedures whose value is really established, and to delineate those that still require validation.'

Sitting isolated at the centre of these, often dubious, precautions is the patient. Horton and Parker (1997) cite Coleman's (1987) description of isolation as a bitter, toxic and costly pill, and of other studies describing the cognitive and sensory disturbance experienced by patients in isolation. Knowles' small study (1993) found that, while some patients valued the privacy the situation provided, expressions of neglect, isolation, stigmatization and loneliness were common. The author also found that while nurses could describe their patient's responses fairly accurately, . . . 'their ability to alter practice to meet the needs of these patients appeared constrained by time, the physical environment, fear of infection and the limitations of describing nursing interventions primarily in terms of physical care'.

It could, therefore, be argued that the isolation policies that form one of the cornerstones of infection control practice are not so much a distillation of science, but rather a social construct reflecting the beliefs and values of those who write the policy, the culture in which the policy is implemented, and the physical and financial constraints of the organization. Evidence for this assertion lies in differences in isolation policies across the UK and in the many ways that national guidelines (such as those for methicillin-resistant *Staphylococcus aureus*) (MRSA) are interpreted for local use. In the case of MRSA examples include: masks are worn, masks are not worn; single rooms are used, single rooms are not used; staff are screened, staff are not screened.

The reality of the situation is that those who have, or can get, the kind of resources Williams (1970) wrote about do one thing, whereas and those without similar resources do something else. Barrett *et al.* (1993) compared MRSA policies in three neighbouring health authorities and concluded that the experience of those who committed the least resources was no different from those who committed the most resources. This has to be puzzling for clinical staff, including infection control practitioners, who move between hospitals. They inevitably ask why one hospital does this and another does that, when both are dealing with the same organism.

A new facet was added to the isolation conundrum in the 1980s with the advent of HIV, and recognition that it could be spread by blood-to-blood contact. Although there were dissenting voices, there was recognition that staff were at risk and that potentially HIV-positive people could not necessarily be identified from their case histories. A new strategy was needed to protect staff from bloodborne infections. The concept of universal precautions, i.e. a policy universally applied to all patients irrespective of disease status, was developed in the USA (Centres for Disease Control, 1986). These aimed to prevent exposure to blood. Following seroconversion in health care workers exposed to blood on non-intact skin and mucous membranes, universal precautions (UP) were modified to take this into account (Centres for Disease Control, 1987, 1988). This approach was tacitly accepted in the UK in 1990 (UK Health Departments).

Universal precautions and the Department of Health guidelines were not universally welcomed. The belief that HIV-positive or hepatitis B-positive people could be recognized, and dealt with differently, persisted. This was not unexpected when isolation precautions had always been diagnosis driven. However, the concept of UP found favour with many clinicians. Others felt that gloves put an unacceptable barrier between the clinician and patient; yet others felt that clinicians should not be afraid to use bare hands. Another group felt that gloves impeded their manual dexterity, and placed them more at risk.

Meanwhile, infection control practitioners in Seattle had spent three years studying a system they called body substance isolation (BSI) (Lynch *et al.*, 1987). BSI focused on the use of gloves for contact with moist body substances, irrespective of disease status. In effect, Lynch and colleagues stood isolation precautions on their head and tried to close the gap between acquiring an infection and the diagnosis of infection. Some evidence exists that BSI, or a modification of it to include gowns, can prevent some infections (e.g. Weinstein and Kabias, 1981; Leclair *et al.*, 1987; Klein *et al.*, 1989). While the evidence is not robust, BSI had a rational appeal. As a system, it had some weaknesses. It did not include handwashing after glove removal unless the hands were soiled. There is evidence that hands can become contaminated when gloves are worn or when the gloves are removed. It did not take sufficient account of droplet or airborne spread, or of the importance of dry skin and the environment as reservoirs. There was also the risk of staff protecting themselves at the expense of patients, e.g. not changing gloves between patients.

Resistance to UP and BSI was both cultural and financial. Beliefs about the ability to recognize patients with bloodborne viruses, and that these patients were unlikely to be found outside metropolitan areas, persisted. Staff who wore gloves were sometimes regarded as weak or inadequate practitioners. Increased use of gloves was claimed to be too expensive, although the comparison between the various costs was seldom made explicit, e.g. limited use of gloves which left expensively trained staff unprotected, or wider use of gloves which gave them a measure of protection. These views continue to be expressed, though less often. There has to be some sympathy with them since, like so much else in the field of isolation, robust scientific evidence is lacking. On the other hand, the outcome of many infection control activities is demonstrated by a negative, e.g. because we did this, infections did not happen. The outcome, had UP and BSI not been used, will never be known.

In the UK, Wilson and Breedon (1990) described the concept of universal infection control precautions (UICP) which brought together UP and BSI, but set them within the context of the UK health care system. The concept was widely accepted. It is now hard to find any health care setting, from GP and dental surgeries to tertiary referral centres, where UICP in some form is not practised. Whether the form adopted is always the most effective is unknown.

In 1996, the Centres for Disease Control synthesized the major features of UP and BSI as Standard Precautions (HICPAC, 1996). These are the first, and most important, tier of their latest isolation guidelines, and are intended to be applied irrespective of diagnosis or presumed infection status. The second tier of transmission-based precautions includes Airborne, Droplet and Contact Precautions. This new approach takes into account the importance of emerging multi-drug-resistant organisms such as tuberculosis and vancomycin-resistant enterococci. It is in the introduction of these guidelines that HICPAC makes the statement quoted earlier on gaps in knowledge.

The first section of this chapter has set isolation precautions in context, and recognized explicitly that a scientific basis for precautions is often lacking. It has also recognized, albeit controversially, that the development and content of individual isolation policies has a social, cultural, organizational and financial component. To be even more explicit, many infection control practitioners know that certain things can or cannot be written into isolation policies because a powerfully-placed individual wishes it so. Moreover, it has recognized that the patient's needs may not be considered, or may be overridden, by the isolation policy and the perceived need to isolate a germ. Nurses may feel powerless to alter their practice to meet the patient's needs. This is an important dimension to bear in mind when developing isolation policies, since all nurses are subject to the UKCC Code of Professional Conduct, which places the patient at the centre of nursing practice. Isolation may sometimes conflict with this. Horton and

Table 7.1	Routes of transmission of infectious diseases
Route	Example of infection
Airborne	
Droplet nuclei	Chicken-pox, measles, pulmonary tuberculosis
Skin scales	Staphylococcal skin lesions
Droplets	Invasive haemophilus and meningococcal infections
	Gram-negative bacilli or Staph. aureus infection (respiratory tract)
	Mycoplasma pneumoniae, whooping cough, diphtheria, rubella, mumps, streptococcal pharyngitis, influenza, adenovirus infection, RSV
Contact	
Wound	Infected discharging wounds or abscesses, varicose ulcers, pressure sores, (MRSA, VRE)
Secretion/	Conjunctivitis, herpes simplex and herpes zoster
excretion	Urinary tract infection
Faecal oral	Shigella, salmonella, E.coli 0157, rotavirus, Cl. difficile, campylobacter, cholera, hepatitis A
Blood	HBV, HCV, HIV, haemorrhagic viral infections

Parker (1997) neatly summarize the ethical dilemmas inherent in decision-making on isolation.

The sections that follow accept the realities set out above. They also draw on the concept of a chain of infection, in particular the source (Chapter 2), the host (Chapter 3) and transmission (Chapters 3 and 8). Examples of modes of transmission of infections are shown in Table 7.1. However, not all these have a single mode of spread and in some instances there is even no general agreement, e.g. between the relative importance of airborne, droplet or contact spread.

Approaches to isolation

Current isolation has three broad approaches:

- The first might be called the conventional approach. This has a detailed written policy, which is activated by clinical or laboratory diagnosis of infection.
- Universal Infection Control Precautions plus additional precautions activated by clinical or laboratory diagnosis of infection spread by the airborne route or droplets, and some infectious spread by contact.
- Risk assessment, which includes the UICP method plus a judgement on additional precautions based on a range of factors including the patient's abilities and needs, the care setting and the level of risk posed by the organism to other patients and staff.

The divisions between these three approaches are somewhat artificial, and all have advantages and disadvantages. Risk assessment underpins the conventional approach, but judgement on risk is made by a group of experts and codified into a policy which is then applied by rote. It has the advantage of being clear-cut and detailed.

As a written policy, it has a legal status. It does not require thought or judgement by staff who may be inexperienced. On the other hand, it does not let staff tailor isolation precautions to the needs and abilities of the patient. A case history illustrates some of the disadvantages. A particular hospital's policy required staff to wear masks when caring for patients colonized or infected by MRSA. One colonized patient was profoundly deaf, but an accomplished lip-reader. The care team was told not to vary the policy for this patient. This distressed both the patient and the care team, so they decided to ignore that aspect of the isolation policy. So far as the staff were aware, there were no adverse consequences. Thus the policy, and the clinical judgement of the infection control team, were called into question.

The UICP method requires clinical staff to wear, and change, gloves in clearly defined circumstances. They are also required to make a risk assessment of when additional protective clothing is required. Additional precautions came into play for infections spread by droplets or the airborne route, and some spread by contact, e.g. antibiotic-resistant organism. Thus, decision-making is shared between a group of experts and the care team. There is clearly more room for error and it has been argued that it is unfair to transfer responsibility for decisions for containing infection to staff who may be inexperienced. It also requires greater input from the infection control team in the form of teaching, advice, support and monitoring. The fact that this approach has been widely adopted may indicate something about the value of partnership with the care team. On the other hand, the system is easily subverted. Anecdotes abound on the misuse of gloves to protect staff alone rather than patients and staff.

Risk assessment and risk management are integral parts of human activity. In recent years risk assessment has become more explicit in health care, and its impact on infection control has been profound. Instead of relying on a single, catch-all policy, infection control teams have moved to a process of algorithms, flow charts or other decision-making tools which allow a range of decisions in a range of circumstances. It is far from being an easy option, not least because much of infection control is logical or rational, rather than evidence based. However, in relation to isolation it places the patient, as a unique individual, at the heart of the decision-making process. It avoids over-isolation and inappropriate use of single rooms. As with UICP, it increases the need for training, support and monitoring but it has a degree of future proofing that other approaches lack.

Ongoing reform of the NHS is blurring the boundaries between hospital and community, and changing how, where and by which method health care is delivered. The conventional isolation policy was designed for different wards, buildings, staffing structures, technology, expectations and sometimes even different diseases. The nature of risk assessment is able to encompass these changes provided, and it is an important provision, that leadership of this immensely complex process continues to be given to infection control specialists.

Aim of isolation

The aim of isolation is to protect individuals, groups and society from infectious diseases. It is the last line of defence in a range of public health and health care measures intended to promote health and prevent disease. Isolation in relation to hospital-acquired infection (HAI) occupies a unique niche in that the infection requiring some form of isolation is a consequence of a health care intervention. Within HAI, colonization by antibiotic-resistant organisms, often recognized only on selective laboratory examination or screening, presents its own unique problems. Therefore, isolation precautions, however they are delivered, take place within a context of other measures, e.g. immunization and vaccination, health promotion, and guidelines on prevention of HAI.

The aim of isolation precautions may, therefore, be defined as reducing the risk of the spread of infection, before and after diagnosis, to susceptible individuals, including health care workers. (For protective isolation see p. 198.)

Universal infection control precautions

However controversial it may once have been, the UICP method is now probably the most important method of protecting patients and staff from infection. Used wisely, it can limit the need for single room isolation. The precise components of what constitutes UICP may vary between trusts. Effective infection control has always involved certain universal precautions, e.g. handwashing, care in handling linen and waste, etc., and the main difference in the present requirements is that gloves are worn to protect staff when handling blood and body fluids in addition to known contaminated materials. Ward *et al.* (1997) list the common essential components:

• prevent blood/body substance contact with non-intact skin and mucous membranes
• minimize blood/body substance contact with intact skin
• prevent sharps injuries
• immunize staff against hepatitis B
• prevent contaminated items being used between patients.

In the USA, the Hospital Infection Control Practices Advisory Committee (HICPAC) (1996) has synthesized the major features of blood and body fluid precautions and body substance isolation as standard precautions and applies them to all patients receiving care in hospitals, regardless of their diagnosis or presumed infection status. In the UK, UICP fulfils much the same function.

Additional precautions

Patients diagnosed as or suspected of having highly transmissible or epidemiologically important infections, particularly those spread by droplets, the airborne route or contact, may need additional precautions. The main additional requirement for airborne, droplet and some types of contact spread (e.g. for antibiotic-resistant organisms) is a single room (HICPAC, 1996).

Some hospitals may prefer to continue with the original category system of standard or contact, respiratory (or airborne), enteric and protective (Ayliffe *et al.*, 1992; Damani, 1997). Coloured cards indicating the category are still commonly used. The strict isolation category is rarely required and the blood category has usually been replaced by universal precautions.

Cross-infection in our own isolation ward of 12 cubicles has been minimal over more than 20 years and a few basic procedures have been strictly implemented (Ayliffe *et al.*, 1979). These are as follows:

- use of single cubicles with a washhand basin and extractor fans for airborne infections
- keeping doors of cubicles closed
- handwashing/disinfection after contact with patients or their immediate surroundings
- wearing plastic aprons for handling patients
- wearing gloves for contact with potentially contaminated body fluids or materials
- care in disposal of used linen, needles and other clinical waste and heat disinfection of crockery and cutlery.

Gloves are now worn when handling blood and all body fluids. If splashng with blood is likely, a mask and eye protection may be used, but this is rarely required.

The elements of UICP and additional aspects are considered in greater detail in the following sections or chapters.

Single room

A single room with the door shut is intended to prevent the transmission of organisms spread by the airborne route, and to prevent gross contamination of the environment outside of the room with certain organisms spread by contact. An extraction system (e.g. a window fan) providing 8–10 air changes per hour is desirable to prevent airborne spread. A more expensive extraction system with filtration may be preferred if highly drug-resistant tuberculosis is a problem. For non-airborne infections requiring a single room, it is still preferable to keep the door closed, but for certain patients leaving the door open may be considered. It is often difficult to define the relative importance of airborne droplet and contact spread in many infections. Confinement to a single room can be an unpleasant experience. While it is necessary to restrict the patient, it can also discourage staff from entering the room. The patient can feel deprived of human contact, so a single room should not be used if airborne transmission is unlikely or if there is little risk of heavy environmental contamination.

Patients often say that having to call a nurse to a single room makes them feel as if they are being a nuisance. Staff should, therefore, be encouraged to visit frequently and when possible spend time with the patients. Large windows, a tidy well-decorated room and a television and radio all help to reduce the feeling of isolation.

Table 7.2   Recovery of *Staphylococcus aureus* and Gram-negative bacilli from nurses' uniforms after wearing cotton gowns or plastic aprons on an isolation ward*

No. of colony-forming units per contact plate (25 cm²)	Cotton gowns		Plastic aprons	
	Front (n = 133)	Shoulder (n = 118)	Front (n = 166)	Shoulder (n = 166)
Staphylococcus aureus				
0	89 (66.9%)	89 (75.4%)	118 (75.1%)	134 (80.7%)
1–10	43 (32.3%)	29 (24.6%)	46 (23.7%)	30 (18.1%)
11–50	1 (0.7%)	0	2 (1.2%)	1 (0.6%)
51+	0	0	0	1 (0.6%)
Gram-negative bacilli				
0	126 (94.7%)	112 (94.9%)	162 (97.6%)	163 (98.2%)
1–10	7 (5.3%)	6 (5.1%)	3 (1.8%)	3 (1.8%)
11–50	0	0	1 (0.6%)	0
51+	0	0	0	0

* From Babb *et al.* (1983) *J. Hosp. Infect.*, 4, 149–157.

Aprons

Transmission of organisms from clothing of staff is possible but is not a major problem (Table 7.2). Heavy contamination of protective clothing was uncommon in our study, and Gram-negative bacilli were infrequently isolated. However, it is rational to protect uniforms when infected material is being handled. The area at waist height is most often contaminated, but may extend to lower or higher levels depending on the procedure. An impermeable plastic apron offers better protection than a cotton gown, although the latter is often preferred by medical staff. It is uncommon for the shoulder area of the uniform to become contaminated, even when lifting a patient, but long sleeves should be rolled up.

It is difficult to understand the rationale for keeping gowns hanging outside the room, since this will neither contain contamination inside the room nor prevent transfer outside. If the gown is intended to prevent uniforms becoming contaminated, it does so by itself becoming contaminated. It presents no risk to the infected patient because he already has the disease. The relative lack of evidence for the spread of infection by this route indicates the low risk of infection attached to protective clothing. However, clothing may transfer staphylococci from the rooms of heavy dispersers (Hambraeus, 1973).

Masks

At one time it was common practice to wear conventional masks for many ward procedures. It is now recognized that this practice contributes little to patient or staff safety on the wards (Taylor, 1980). The rationale for wearing a mask is either to protect the patient from the staff or the staff from the patient. If a health care worker has a cold, a sore throat or influenza, he/she should be off duty, not wearing a mask. *Staph. aureus* is unlikely to be dispersed in the air in large numbers directly from the nose of a carrier. It is more likely to be spread by improper use of a mask, i.e. handling the mask, followed by handling the patient without washing the hands first. Masks are no substitute for good technique and careful handwashing. There is an area of uncertainty as regards the use of masks by staff dressing burns or large open wounds, and for certain procedures, e.g. lumbar puncture and bone marrow biopsy. While there is no great evidence that use of a mask contributes to preventing infection in these circumstances, some authorities may still recommend their use. There is also no good evidence of the protective effect in staff of wearing a conventional mask against the acquisition of respiratory viral infections. However, masks may sometimes be recommended for staff in close contact with infections spread by droplets (HICPAC, 1996).

As regards the common childhood fevers, non-immune staff should not be allowed to care for such patients. There may be some reason for wearing a mask during the first 48 h of specific treatment for meningococcal meningitis, although by the time a bacteriological diagnosis is made it may be rather late to do so, and there is little evidence of spread to hospital staff. Specific antibiotic prophylaxis is more appropriate. If a mask is thought necessary, it should be an efficient filter type.

Open pulmonary tuberculosis, suspected or diagnosed, presents specific problems, particularly if a multi-drug-resistant tuberculosis (MDRTB) strain is suspected. Conventional masks offer limited protection. Staff working with vulnerable groups may wish to use high-efficiency filtration masks. There is some controversy about the value of these masks, but it seems pointless to deny their use to staff who may be working with MDRTB. It is better that staff are trained in the use of the masks and use them according to a mutually agreed protocol.

The use of BCG to protect tuberculin-negative staff has been generally successful in the UK and few acquisitions have been reported in hospitals where pulmonary tuberculosis has been treated, but these infections have been mainly caused by sensitive strains.

Handwashing

As stated in Chapters 5, 6 and 11, handwashing is the most important method of preventing the spread of infection by contact. In our study on an isolation ward, there was no cross-infection when non-medicated bar soap, chlorhexidine detergent or 70% alcohol was used. Bacterial counts from finger impressions showed little difference (Table 7.3) between the three regimes, although Gram-negative bacilli were less after the use of 70% alcohol. It is more important to ensure that hands are actually washed or disinfected than to worry about the choice of agents. Nevertheless, alcohol rubs are convenient and more effective than washing when tested in the laboratory and their use should be encouraged after contact with infected patients.

Gloves

Gloves are used for a variety of reasons:

- as a protective barrier to prevent contamination when touching blood, body fluids, secretions, excretions, mucous membranes and non-intact skin

Table 7.3   Influence of soap and antiseptics on the transient hand carriage of nurses in an isolation ward*

Range of cfu[†] per sample	Percentage of samples					
	Chlorhexidine detergent		Bar soap		70% alcohol	
	Staph. aureus	GNB[‡]	Staph. aureus	GNB	Staph. aureus	GNB
1 000 000	0	0	0	2	0	0
10 000–1 000 000	5	10	4	12	8	1
200–10 000	12	11	8	9	13	2
< 200	83	79	88	77	79	97

* From Ayliffe et al. (1988) J. Hosp. Infect., 11, 226–243.[†]cfu = colony-forming units.[‡]GNB = Gram-negative bacilli.

- to protect the patient from the health care worker's normal or transient flora
- to facilitate manipulation of sterile equipment
- to prolong the effect of hand disinfection.

Gloves must be changed after each patient contact, and at the end of each procedure. Hands should be washed after removing the gloves. Hands may be contaminated during glove removal or through inapparent defects or tears. The gloves themselves should not be washed. Non-sterile gloves should be used when handling potentially contaminated material.

The gloves should be of good quality, well fitting and stored in dispenser packs which prevent contamination of the contents when a glove is removed. Latex allergy is increasingly recognized as a problem for both staff and patients. Good-quality, non-latex gloves should be available in these circumstances.

Although the UICP method is now generally accepted in the UK and many other countries and it is accepted that the use of gloves may be better than no handwashing, the effectiveness of using gloves as a substitute for handwashing has not been demonstrated.

Overshoes

In operating theatres, where patients are particularly vulnerable and contamination needs to be kept to a minimum, it is rational to wear different shoes within the theatre suite (see Chapter 16). However, there is no such requirement in isolation nursing. The floor is not a source of infection so long as the patients are nursed in bed, and equipment that falls to the floor is decontaminated before reuse. In one reported incident, the probable cause of an outbreak of *Pseudomonas* infection in a renal unit was the use of overshoes. People entering the unit were required to wear overshoes and in putting them on, the hands were contaminated with *Pseudomonas* organisms from the floor. Patients and equipment were then handled without adequate handwashing. The method of spread was clearly by contact associated with poor handwashing, but this was secondary to the unnecessary use of overshoes. Any *Pseudomonas* organisms would otherwise have stayed harmlessly on the floor.

Equipment
Whether a patient is being isolated or not, equipment must be sterilized or properly decontaminated before reuse, or it should be single use. In the case of suspected spongiform encephalopathy, equipment likely to have been in contact with the causative agent is quarantined until a diagnosis is made. If confirmed, the equipment is destroyed. However, if the items of equipment are expensive, and not in contact with the CNS, e.g. gastroscopes, the problem of disposal or decontamination should be discussed with the infection control team (see Chapter 12).

Crockery and cutlery
Lack of evidence for spread by this route may indicate that it is relatively unimportant. Decontamination in a dishwasher with a final rinse temperature of 80°C is the method of choice. Disposable crockery and cutlery should only be needed if there is a fault in the dishwasher or for certain infections, e.g. enteric, if a dishwasher is not available.

Bathing
Bath-water contains large numbers of organisms which are redistributed over the skin and contaminate the towel and environment. Showers are preferable to baths, although environmental contamination still occurs. The bath or shower should be cleaned with a non-abrasive chlorine-releasing agent before and after use.

The bath or shower is an unlikely route of spread of droplet or airborne infection. Patients with infected lesions, urinary tract or enteric infection may benefit from the addition of a disinfectant to the bath-water. Patients who require enhanced contact precautions, where staphylococci rather than Gram-negative bacteria are the main problem, may benefit from the use of chlorhexidine detergent applied to damp skin, then rinsed off. Household salt may still be added to bath water – in the quantities in which it is used, it does not act as a disinfectant.

Aromatherapy oils are gaining popularity with patients and carers alike. In the concentrated form, many oils are microbicidal *in vitro*. They are unlikely to retain this properly when diluted in bath-water.

Patients' wash bowls have been implicated in at least one ward outbreak of infection. A bowl that is inadequately decontaminated before use will still be contaminated by organisms from the previous patient. The organisms most likely to be found are Gram-negative bacteria. Cleaning and thorough drying will reduce their numbers.

Caps
It is difficult to understand the rationale for the use of caps outside the operating theatre. There may be a slight possibility of some transient carriage of *Staph. aureus* on the hair, acquired from a patient with skin disease, possibly during bed-making when large numbers of organisms were dispersed. Provided that the hair is kept clean and tidy, this would seem to be a

minimal risk, not justifying the use of caps. If a member of staff has a skin lesion, including one of the scalp, this requires treatment and possibly sick leave, not the use of protective clothing.

Needles and sharp instruments ('sharps')
Sharp instruments must be disposed of safely, into an approved container by the user, and as close to the point of use as possible. It is worth noting that most injuries to laundry handlers are from 'sharps'. Porters removing waste are particularly at risk from needles inadvertently discarded into plastic bags.

Specimens
Laboratory staff are at risk of acquiring infection, since they handle material from infected patients and may well make the first diagnosis of infection. However, the incidence of laboratory-acquired infection is low. Portering staff are also at some slight risk from contamination of the outside of specimen containers. It is a principle of the UICP method that all specimens and request forms be transported in dual-compartment plastic bags.

Charts
Charts are handled by a variety of people, and it is therefore assumed that they present a greater risk than is usually the case. However, the size of the risk depends on the diligence of handwashing. When a patient requires single room isolation, the charts are more likely to be handled by clean hands, if they are kept outside the room.

Mattress covers and duvets
In general, mattresses and pillows have impermeable covers and can be adequately decontaminated by cleaning with detergent and water. This also applies to duvets contained within an impermeable cover. If disinfection is required, a chlorine-releasing agent should be used, or 70% alcohol (see page 117). Phenolics should not be used as they damage some types of impermeable fabrics. Duvets, other than those encased in an impermeable fabric, should be capable of being laundered.

Visitors
Generous visiting times often lead to claims of increased infection risks, although evidence for this is lacking. Visitors are important for any patient, particularly for patients in single room isolation. Visitors should be advised about handwashing. If they are contributing to the patient's care, as might be the case for a child, they should observe the same precautions as staff. In general, visitors who have an infectious disease, or who are themselves vulnerable to infection, should be advised about the risks and encouraged not to visit. However, this is a very difficult area and should not be the subject of hard-and-fast rules. Risk assessment must be used, taking into account the emotional and social needs of both patient and visitors. The final decision must rest with the patient and his/her family. The task of the care team and the infection control team is to manage the risk and respect the patient's autonomy.

Spillage of body substances
Spillages should be dealt with at once by covering them with absorbent paper towels, cleaning them with detergent and water, and disposal of the debris as clinical waste. Where the surface will withstand it, a chlorine-releasing agent should be used after cleaning (see Chapter 11).

Staff training

New approaches to isolation require an informed workforce and an investment in ongoing training. Conventional approaches require staff to follow a set of rules. They are now required to think about isolation, just as they think about other elements of their practice. New approaches offer greater opportunities for prevention, and for the efficient use of single rooms. Both depend on a hospital-wide commitment and training.

Patient placement

Conventional approaches to isolation consigned infected or colonized patients to a single room. The availability of single rooms, and the pressure on them for other clinical reasons, is such that other solutions to containing infection have to be found. These solutions often depend on seeing the patient as a sentient individual, capable of rational thought, able to contribute to his/her own care and the protection of others. There are many occasions when patients who are willing and able to comply with simple rules can be nursed in bays or open wards. There are also occasions when patients who are confined to bed can be nursed in bays or open wards, provided that staff adhere to the rules. A single room should not be the alternative to involving the patient or to staff compliance with protocols.

A more recent practice that impacts on alternatives to single room isolation is the practice of moving patients between wards during a single admission. In a recent study (Glynn *et al.*, 1997), five to seven moves were not uncommon in some trusts. This practice has a negative impact on measures to prevent, control and contain infection, and it should be avoided.

Summary

This chapter has addressed new and emerging concepts of isolation precautions, and UICP. It recognizes that the patient is the central figure and that care should be directed to meeting patient needs and drawing on his/her abilities. There has to be a balance between containing the organism for the wider good and minimum disruption to the care and recovery of the infected or colonized person. This also reflects the emphasis on evidence-based clinical practice. The Department of Health, Royal Colleges and professional societies produce valuable clinical guidelines. The Infection Control Nurses' Association of the British Isles regularly produces a book listing these, together with many useful references. National infection control guidelines are in preparation.

References and further reading

Ayliffe, G.A.J., Babb, J.R., Taylor, L.J. and Wise, R. (1979). A unit for source and protective isolation in a general hospital. *Br. Med. J.*, **2**, 461–465.

Ayliffe, G.A.J., Babb, J.R., Davies, J.G. and Lilly, H.A. (1988). Hand disinfection: a comparison of various agents in laboratory and ward studies. *J. Hosp. Infect.*, **11**, 226–243.

Ayliffe, G.A.J., Lowbury, E.J.L., Geddes, A.M. and Williams, J.D. (1992) *Control of Hospital Infection. A Practical Handbook*, 3rd edn, London, Chapman and Hall.

Babb, J.R., Davies, J.G. and Ayliffe, G.A.J. (1983) Contamination of protective clothing and nurses' uniforms in an isolation ward. *J. Hosp. Infect.*, **4**, 149–157.

Barrett, S.P., Teare, E.L. and Sage, R. (1993) Methicillin-resistant *Staphylococcus aureus* in three adjacent Health Districts in South-East England 1986–1991. *J. Hosp. Infect.*, **24**, 313–325.

Centres for Disease Control (1986) Recommendations for preventing transmission of infection with human T-lymphotropic virus type III/lymphadenopathy-associated virus during invasive procedures. *MMWR*, **35**, 221–223.

Centres for Disease Control (1987) Recommendations for prevention of HIV transmission in health-care settings. *MMWR*, **36**(2S), 1S–18S.

Centres for Disease Control (1988) Update: universal precautions for prevention of transmission of human immunodeficiency virus, hepatitis B virus, and other bloodborne pathogens in health-care settings. *MMWR*, **37**, 377–382 and 387–388.

Damani, N.N. (1997) *Manual of Infection Control Procedures*, London, Greenwich Medical Media.

Gammon, J. (1998) Analysis of the stressful effects of hospitalisation and source isolation on coping and psychological construct. *Int. J. Nurs. Pract.*, **4**, 84–96.

Garner, J.S. and Hierholzer, W.J. (1993) Controversies in isolation policies and practices. In *Prevention and Control of Nosocomial Infections*, 2nd edn (R.P. Wenzel ed.) Baltimore, Williams and Wilkins, pp.70–81.

Glynn, A., Ward, V., Wilson, J. *et al.* (1997) *Hospital-acquired Infection. Surveillance Policies and Practice*, London, Public Health Laboratory Service.

Hambraeus, A. (1973) Transfer of *Staph. aureus* via nurses' uniforms. *J. Hyg. (Camb.)*, **71**, 799–814.

HICPAC (1996) Guideline for isolation precautions in hospital. *Infect. Control Hosp. Epidemiol.*, **17**(1), 53–80.

Horton, R. and Parker, L. (1997) *Informed Infection Control Practice*, Edinburgh, Churchill Livingstone.

Klein, B.S., Perloff, W.H. and Maki, D.G. (1989) Reduction of nosocomial infection during paediatric intensive care by protective isolation. *New Engl. J. Med.*, **320**, 1714–1721.

Knowles, H.E. (1993) The experience of infectious patients in isolation. *Nurs. Times*, **89**(30), 53–56.

Leclair, J.M., Freeman, J., Sullivan, B.F., Crowley, C.M. and Goldman, D.A. (1987) Prevention of nosocomial respiratory syncytial virus infections through compliance with gown and glove isolation precautions. *New Engl. J. Med.*, **317**, 329–334.

Lynch, P., Jackson, M.M., Cummings, M.J. and Stamm, W.E. (1987) Rethinking the role of isolation practices in the prevention of nosocomial infections. *Ann. Intern. Med.*, **107**, 243–246.

Taylor, L. (1980) Are face masks necessary in operating theatres and wards? *J. Hosp. Infect.*, **1**, 173–174.

UK Health Departments (1998) *Guidance for Clinical Health Care Workers: Protection Against Infections with Blood-borne Viruses*, London, HMSO.

Ward, V., Wilson, J., Taylor, L. *et al.* (1997) *Preventing Hospital-acquired Infection: Clinical Guidelines*, London, Public Health Laboratory Service.

Weinstein, R.A. and Kabias, S.A. (1981) Strategies for prevention and control of multiple drug-resistant nosocomial infection. *Am. J. Med.*, **70**, 449–454.

Williams, R.E.O. (1970) Changing perspectives in hospital infection. In *Proceedings of the International Conference on Nosocomial Infections*, Centers for Disease Control, 3–6, August, 1970, Chicago/American Hospital Association, 1971, pp.1–10.

Wilson, J. and Breedon, P. (1990) Universal precautions. *Nurs. Times*, **86**, 67–70.

8

The hospital environment

Introduction

The hospital environment includes all the physical surroundings of patients and staff, i.e. structures, fittings, fixtures, furnishings, equipment and supplies. The microbiological ecology of the environment is influenced by the persons present and their activities. It is the responsibility of all health carers and infection control practitioners to ensure that the environment and the activities carried out within it do not put the hospital community at risk. (Ayliffe *et al.*, 1976; Collins, 1988).

Any environment can pose an infection hazard to highly susceptible individuals, but the principal requirement is to ensure that the majority of patients are at no greater risk than they would be elsewhere and that we identify and minimize or eliminate environmentally associated risks, particularly to those who are most vulnerable.

The need to control surface and airborne transmission should be considered at an early stage, particularly if new building works are planned or the purchase of new equipment is being considered. It may be difficult or impossible to make major changes at a later date.

Rendering the environment safe may involve the provision of cleaning, disinfection, sterilization and ventilation facilities. Each of these methods is likely to be progressively more expensive and cost must therefore be related to infection risk. To choose the most appropriate method of decontamination requires a knowledge of specific sources and routes of transmission (see Chapter 3). Collaboration is therefore necessary between those providing and receiving health care and particularly those responsible for decontamination, maintenance and infection control. Control measures should be based on sound infection control principles which can be summarized as follows:

1. The environment should be hostile to the multiplication of pathogenic micro-organisms, i.e. clean, dry and well ventilated.
2. Susceptible sites, e.g. wounds, and particularly vulnerable patients (immunosuppressed) should be protected by the application of a suitable dressing or nursed in a single room within an isolation unit.
3. Where possible, the immune response of a susceptible host (patient or member of staff) should be increased by immunization, e.g. HBV vaccination for staff working in an accident and emergency or dialysis unit.

4.   Infectious material should be adequately contained and/or removed. Surfaces or items likely to make contact with a susceptible site, or that are invasive, should be cleaned and disinfected or sterilized to prevent the transfer of infection.

Consideration of these principles can assist in the identification of potentially high-risk situations, e.g.:

1.   Pathogens may grow where there is spillage of blood, pus, urine, vomit or faeces, unless it is removed promptly and both the spillage and cleaning materials are disposed of safely.
2.   Raw meat, waste food, used cleaning materials or wet equipment are usually heavily contaminated with Gram-negative bacilli which may include intestinal, wound and urinary pathogens, e.g. *Pseudomonas aeruginosa* and *Salmonella* spp.
3.   Bathrooms, toilets and sluice rooms are moist areas and are often badly ventilated. These conditions may be conducive to the survival and growth of Gram-negative bacilli.
4.   Equipment likely to come into contact with a break in the skin or mucous membranes, or to be inserted into sterile body cavities, requires sterilization, e.g. dressings, surgical instruments, sutures, catheters, parenteral fluids and implants.
5.   Materials that have been in contact with body fluids or patients with specific infections may require particular care in handling, transportation and disposal, e.g. soiled dressings or linen.
6.   The immediate environment of a patient suffering from an unusually virulent infection, or a specified communicable disease, may require additional decontamination measures to ensure it is safe for reuse by another patient.
7.   Additional resources may be required to make the immediate environment safe for use by a highly susceptible patient, e.g. units for the treatment of leukaemics and other heavily immunosuppressed patients, operating theatres, intensive care and special care baby units.

Some surfaces, e.g. walls, floors, furniture, fixtures and fittings, are unlikely to come into prolonged or intimate contact with a susceptible site and are a low infection risk. These surfaces rarely require more than periodic cleaning. Pathogens are unlikely to be present on dry surfaces in sufficient numbers to cause infection or, if present, to reach a susceptible site on the patient.

In high-risk situations, more frequent cleaning may be required and surfaces, furnishings and fittings should be chosen which are easy to clean and dry and will withstand frequent and thorough cleaning without excessive deterioration. The complete removal of all micro-organisms is not practical or desirable, except for 'high-risk' items such as surgical instruments.

The unnecessary use of chemical disinfectants, harsh cleaning materials or even excessive amounts of water can shorten the life of environmental surfaces. An example is the frequent cleaning and disinfection of mattress covers with phenolic disinfectants which may damage the waterproofing and allow moisture to penetrate, enabling *Ps. aeruginosa* and other Gram-negative bacilli to grow in the foam under the cover (Lilly *et al.*, 1982). These organisms may then spread from the mattress to lesions on a patient subsequently occupying the bed. Disinfectants have also been responsible for erosion of terrazzo floors and the hardening and discoloration of plastic floor coverings. Excessive use of water which penetrates joints and coverings may provide sufficient trapped moisture to allow bacteria to grow under the material, causing damage to the underlying structure. Disinfectants may also exert a selective influence on the microbial population. Outbreaks of infection caused by resistant *Ps. aeruginosa* and *Serratia marcescens* have occurred in intensive care units possibly due to the indiscriminate, and often illogical, use of disinfectants and concentrations to which these organisms are resistant. This allows them to grow and reach unusually high numbers.

Another cause for concern with the heavy use of disinfectants are their irritant and sensitizing properties. Most of the more effective environmental and equipment disinfectants, e.g. chlorine-releasing agents, phenols and aldehydes, are irritant and sensitizing to the skin, eyes and respiratory tract. Employers have a responsibility, under the Control of Substances Hazardous to Health Regulations (COSHH), to protect health care workers from unnecessary and unprotected exposure to these agents. Careful consideration should therefore be given to the benefits of using disinfectants. If, having carefully assessed the need, they are used, instruction should be given on how they should be prepared and used so as to protect the user and others which might be exposed. Personal protective equipment, e.g. gloves and apron and some form of ventilation, may be required.

Bacteria cannot grow or survive for long periods on clean dry surfaces and disinfection of environmental surfaces, furniture, fixtures and fittings is rarely required, except following soiling by potentially infectious material, e.g. blood, pus, faeces or urine from patients with transmissible infections. In high-risk areas, the need to select material capable of withstanding frequent and thorough cleaning and disinfection may conflict with its appearance or patient comfort, e.g. carpets. However, this is not a problem in all clinical areas and a balance between infection risk, appearance and ease of maintenance must be achieved.

Air

The numbers of micro-organisms present in air within a room will depend on the number of people occupying that room, their activity and the rate at which particles settle or the air is replaced (Lowbury and Ayliffe, 1982). Bacteria recovered from air samples consist of mainly Gram-positive cocci, e.g. *Staph. epidermidis* originating from the skin of the occupants. Pathogens are usually few and of these *Staph. aureus* is the most likely. *Staph. aureus* can reach large numbers if dispersed from a patient or member of staff with an infected lesion, or particularly from an exfoliative skin condition, e.g. eczema (see Chapter 2). Since contaminated skin squames are relatively heavy they will not usually remain suspended in the air for long periods. Droplets projected from the infected upper respiratory tract may contain a wide variety of organisms and some infections can be spread by this route, e.g. colds, influenza, childhood infectious diseases and tuberculosis, but an infective dose, with some exceptions, is rarely carried more than a metre or two before the droplets settle or the organisms die. However, some bacteria (e.g. tubercle bacilli) and viruses may remain viable in dried droplets (droplet nuclei) and can be transported for considerable distances. Gram-negative bacteria only tend to be found in the air when associated with aerosols generated from contaminated fluids, e.g. from humidifiers, nebulizers and wet cleaning equipment. These tend to die on drying but spread can sometimes occur over relatively long distances, e.g. *Legionella* drift from cooling towers and sprinklers.

In exceptional circumstances, other skin-associated bacteria, e.g. *Staph. epidermidis*, can cause infection, but their source, especially in hospital wards, is more likely to be autogenous transfer from the patient's own skin, e.g. to an intravascular catheterization site.

Mechanical ventilation of wards or dressing stations may be required for comfort but is unlikely to reduce infection rates (Ayliffe, 1974; NHS Estates, 1993a). The 20–25 air changes per hour normally provided in ventilated operating theatres is sufficient for most general surgery and is probably required more to improve comfort than to reduce infection risk. The provision of ultra-clean air can be of value in joint replacement or other implant surgery and may be of value where large incisions remain exposed for long periods, e.g. cardiovascular surgery, but there is no evidence to justify the additional expense for bowel or routine surgery. Nevertheless, an improved method of ventilation should provide maximum protection at the wound site. *Aspergillus fumigatus*, and occasionally other fungal spores, may cause an invasive infection in severely immunocompromised patients (see Chapter 3). It is normally present in the air and is particularly likely to be transmitted during building operations in or close to the hospital. Prevention requires high level air filtration. Dust screens and exhaust ventilation may also be necessary to remove dust, fungal and clostridial spores during reconstruction or fabric renovation work.

Exhaust ventilation, either from the room or from an airlock between the room and corridor, is preferred for source isolation of infected patients. The patients most suited are those with eczema, tuberculosis, viral respiratory infections or those likely to disperse large numbers of multi-resistant strains of staphylococci, e.g. MRSA, from the skin or infected lesions. Some hospitals now have isolation units where single-bedded rooms are equipped with both source and protective isolation facilities (Ayliffe *et al.*, 1979). This is done by supplying each room with a filtered positive pressure air supply at about 7–8 changes per hour. If a patient requires source isolation, an extractor fan is turned on which extracts air more rapidly (e.g. 13–20 changes per hour) than is coming in. This creates a negative pressure within the cubicle (Figure 8.1).

Influence of design

The microbial population of any enclosed space can be influenced by design. An adequate air flow will help to remove micro-organisms as they are dispersed. If the room is inhabited, little can be achieved by temperature

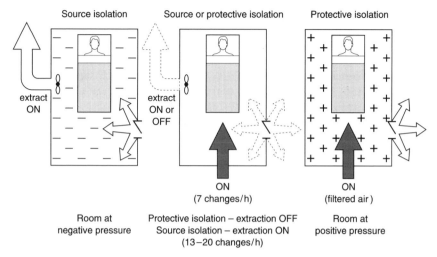

Figure 8.1   Control of airborne infection in isolation wards

control since human pathogens tend to survive well at any temperature in the range acceptable to people. Moisture control is more important since most microbes multiply readily in a moist environment. The provision of surfaces which can easily be kept clean and dry, and on which soil or spillage is readily seen and removed, will reduce infection risk. Bacteria-carrying particles tend to settle on horizontal surfaces and will not readily adhere to smooth vertical surfaces. Heavily textured and moisture-retaining surfaces, and any inaccessible areas where moisture or soil may accumulate, should therefore be avoided in patient treatment areas. However, environmental surfaces are unlikely to be a major infection hazard and in most areas other factors such as cost and appearance may be more relevant.

Floors, carpets and other horizontal surfaces

Bacteria shed by patients and staff will usually be dispersed as skin squames or droplets from the respiratory tract and will tend to be carried on particles more than 10 µm in diameter. Bacteria-carrying particles shed by infected, patients or those carrying multi-resistant strains such as MRSA, and their immediate surroundings, e.g. clothing and bedding, are the greatest risk. In reasonably still air these particles settle fairly rapidly onto horizontal surfaces, usually the floor. After deposition they will tend to remain unless disturbed (Ayliffe *et al.*, 1967). The number of bacteria present on the floor of a busy 30-bedded ward may be quite high, e.g. between 1000 and 2000 colony-forming units per 100 cm^2. The predominant organisms are likely to be *Staph. epidermidis* and other coagulase-negative cocci and diphtheroids present on shed skin squames and *Bacillus* spp. These organisms make up about 99% of the total on a dry ward floor. The only potential pathogens commonly found, but rarely in large numbers, are *Staph. aureus* and *Clostridium perfringens*, but infection risk is small. *Staph. epidermidis* and diphtheroids from inanimate surfaces rarely cause infections. *Staph. aureus* and *Clostridium* spp., although capable of causing infection, are not likely to reach a susceptible site in sufficient numbers to cause infection unless vigorously redistributed into the air, e.g. by sweeping with a broom. Even then, the evidence of hazard is doubtful, particularly with clostridia. Normal movement and air currents have little influence on airborne counts and different types of hard flooring show only minor differences.

Gram-negative bacteria are rare in a dry environment. Their presence is often associated with recent wet cleaning or fluid spillage, but they tend to disappear rapidly as the surface dries. Some organisms survive for longer periods if protected by layers of grease or protein from blood, secretions and excretions.

The behaviour of organisms on soft floor coverings such as carpets is different. Although bacteria are present in larger numbers and survive for longer periods than on hard floors, there is no evidence that they are associated with a greater infection risk. Nevertheless it is still reasonable to minimize potential infection hazard by selecting carpets for use in clinical areas with certain desirable features, e.g. waterproof backing, sealed joints and a short, water repellent, upright and non-absorbent pile (Ayliffe *et al.*, 1974; Collins, 1979). This will ensure the carpet is easily cleaned and dried. Most disinfectants suitable for blood and other body fluid spills damage carpets. However, provided that those responsible for spillage removal wear suitable protective clothing, a compatible detergent is used and the carpet soon dries, odours are unlikely and infection risk is minimal.

Carpets should be vacuumed daily and periodically cleaned with steam/ hot water and vacuum extraction. Absorbent powders may be used on small spills. These can subsequently be removed with a vacuum cleaner.

The decision as to whether or not carpets should be fitted in clinical areas is difficult and is not based entirely on infection control issues. Carpets in areas with frequent and large-volume spillage, e.g. wards for the mentally handicapped, the incontinent, accident and emergency departments and delivery suites, are not recommended as routine cleaning is likely to be inadequate. Problems of smell and staining have resulted in the removal of carpets from some hospitals.

In spite of these maintenance difficulties carpets are still popular with patients as they reduce noise and are more comfortable and homely than hard floor coverings. Should it be decided that carpets are to be fitted in clinical areas, suitable cleaning equipment must be purchased at the same time, spillages dealt with promptly and carpet-compatible cleaning agents used.

In hospital wards, microbial counts from floors tend to remain remarkably static throughout the day, cleaning and disinfection having only a temporary effect on numbers. This is because bacteria tend to be shed at a fairly constant rate by the same group of individuals occupying the room. Factors which affect the rate of dying of bacteria are also reasonably constant, e.g. temperature, ultraviolet light and humidity. Cleaning will rapidly reduce counts by about 80%. The use of a disinfectant can further increase the reduction to 95–99%. However, these organisms are rapidly replaced by continuing dispersal from the occupants of the room and a plateau is reached

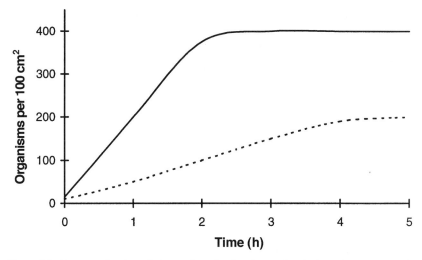

Figure 8.2   Recontamination of floors after cleaning (——, Surgical ward; ----, operating theatre)

in which an equilibrium between deposition and death or removal occurs (Ayliffe *et al.*, 1967). The time taken to establish this equilibrium after cleaning can be as short as 2 h in a large busy ward.

Ventilation delays or prevents settlement of particles and in a theatre with a positive pressure ventilation of 25 changes per hour, 4 h may be necessary before counts return to pre-cleaning levels (Figure 8.2).

While the use of a disinfectant instead of a detergent can increase the reduction in numbers of bacteria by up to 20%, the effect of the additional reduction is so transient that the disadvantages may outweigh the advantages. The disinfectant may be irritant or sensitizing to the user, will add to the cost, possibly increase damage to the surface, may leave behind undesirable residues and can promote a false sense of security. Disinfectants are not, therefore, recommended for routine cleaning.

Occasionally a patient with abnormal skin, e.g. eczema or psoriasis, which has become colonized with *Staph. aureus*, may disperse large numbers of these organisms on skin squames. These patients, i.e. dispersers, may be a substantial risk to others with exposed or uncovered wounds and should be identified and isolated. Dispersal directly from the patient, e.g. during periods of activity, bed making or wound dressing change, is a much greater risk than re-dispersal from horizontal surfaces. Nevertheless, it is sensible to try to eliminate the pathogens in known contaminated spillage and on cleaning equipment more rapidly and completely by using a disinfectant, although it is doubtful that the risk of transfer is greatly reduced. Results obtained from a large survey in the West Midlands showed that the regular use of disinfectants for floor cleaning had no significant effect on wound infection or the nasal acquisition rate of *Staph. aureus* (Collins, 1988).

If it is considered necessary to reduce organisms on the floor surface and on other horizontal surfaces, this can be achieved by reducing the number of occupants in the room, ventilation or increasing the frequency of cleaning.

Accumulation of soil in cracks, joints and corners is unpleasant, but there is little evidence that this is an infection risk. However, joints should preferably be avoided and if unavoidable should be welded or sealed. This prevents an accumulation of organic material which, if moist, would encourage the proliferation of bacteria and unpleasant odours.

Walls and ceilings

Bacteria-containing particles do not readily adhere to walls or attach to ceilings, but may do so if the surface becomes moist, sticky or damaged. Excessive cleaning and the use of harsh chemicals can damage surfaces to the extent that the adhesion of bacteria becomes more likely. However, there is little evidence that walls and ceilings cause infection, even if damaged or contaminated. Bacterial counts from intact vertical wall surfaces are unlikely to exceed one or two colony-forming units per $10 \, cm^2$ and tests carried out in an operating theatre showed no evidence of a build-up over 3–6-month periods (Ayliffe et al., 1967).

Splashes should be cleaned immediately, particularly if they consist of excreta or material known to be contaminated with potential pathogens. Routine cleaning of ward walls at a frequency greater than once a year cannot be justified on infection control grounds. More frequent cleaning of walls of operating theatres and pharmacy clean rooms, e.g. 6 monthly, may be considered desirable, but even in these areas there is little evidence that more frequent cleaning will reduce numbers of bacteria on the wall or in the air. Smooth impervious finishes are preferred in patient treatment areas because they are easier to clean and dry and bacteria will not readily adhere to them, but it is doubtful if, where textured surfaces have been installed, this will greatly increase the infection risk. The space above false ceilings may allow dust to accumulate and can provide harbourage for pests. Where present, this space should be checked on completion of building works to ensure that it has been left clean and not used for discarding unwanted materials. Roof spaces and false ceilings should also be checked to ensure that there is no access for birds and other pests. Perforated ceilings and removable tiles may allow dust and bacterial and fungal spores to fall to the area below, particularly if disturbed during maintenance work. Unless adequately sealed, this type of ceiling is probably undesirable in operating rooms, treatment areas and pharmacy clean rooms.

Fixtures, fittings and furniture

Fixtures and fittings should be designed and constructed so that they are easy to clean and do not accumulate dirt. Electric points and switches likely to be splashed or become wet during cleaning should be of the type that are safe and will not allow moisture penetration. All fixtures and fittings should be listed and included in cleaning schedules.

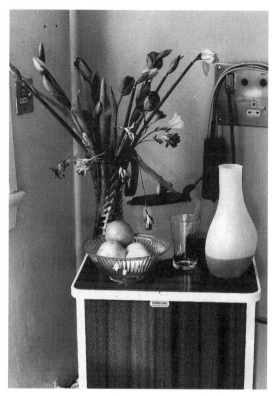

Figure 8.3   Urine bottles as possible source of infection; flowers are an unlikely source

Furniture is a minor infection risk, but should preferably have readily cleanable surfaces, an impervious finish, and be free from ledges which may accumulate dust or retain moisture (Figure 8.3). Furniture should be positioned and designed to prevent dust and dirt accumulating in inaccessible areas below or behind it. It should also be possible to clean it with the equipment provided. Upholstered chairs with foam filling and permeable covers are unsuitable for incontinent patients or those with discharging wounds, as the foam may become contaminated allowing Gram-negative bacteria to proliferate. This would then act as a reservoir of infection and unpleasant odours.

Patient supports, mattresses and pillow and duvet covers described as waterproof or repellent may rapidly become pervious when subjected to regular cleaning and disinfection (Lilly *et al.*, 1982). The manufacturers should be consulted on suitable methods of decontamination and, if covers cannot be removed and laundered, they should not be purchased. Covers should be examined at regular intervals, and stained or worn areas checked to ensure they are impervious to body fluids. The chlorine-releasing agents (i.e. sodium dichloroisocyanurate, NaDCC, or sodium hypochlorite, NaOCl) at 1000 ppm av Cl are currently recommended for mattress covers and supports which cannot be thermally disinfected. Many disinfectants damage fabrics and compatibility should be confirmed with the manufacturers. A wipeover with a neutral detergent followed by drying should be sufficient for routine cleaning.

Sinks, wash-basins and drains

Although sinks and drains are usually contaminated with Gram-negative bacilli, especially *Ps. aeruginosa*, they are infrequently a source of infection (Lowbury *et al.*, 1970; Ayliffe *et al.*, 1974). Sinks and wash-basins should either be sealed to the wall or sufficiently far from the wall to allow access for cleaning. Where sinks or sluices are used for emptying body or cleaning fluids, a splash-back should be fitted which facilitates cleaning and prevents wall damage.

Taps that cause splashing from a shallow bowl or discharge directly into the sink outlet may disperse contaminated aerosols and should be avoided. Sink outlets and U-bends are commonly colonized with large numbers of Gram-negative bacilli and dispersal of them into the clinical environment should be avoided during cleaning and maintenance. Overflows are difficult to clean and rapidly become contaminated. These should be avoided in wash hand basins in high-risk areas as they may become reservoirs of epidemic strains of Gram-negative bacilli. Wash hand basins and scrub sinks designed exclusively for this purpose should have elbow mixer taps and no overflow or plug. The walls of the sink should be designed to deflect water splashes away from those washing their hands. Parts that may become contaminated or colonized with epidemic strains should be easy to remove, clean and replace.

Water supply

Freshly drawn mains water is usually of good microbiological quality and contains very few bacteria. Chlorine-releasing agents are usually added by the water authority and kept at a carefully controlled level which is sufficient to prevent bacterial multiplication (0.5–1 ppm av Cl). When this water is stored in open tanks for long periods, contamination with algae, protozoa, insects, dead birds or their droppings may neutralize the chlorine. If this occurs the small number of bacteria present may proliferate and reach large numbers. While many of the organisms present are not recognized as pathogens, and rarely cause infection, they can contaminate equipment and could cause infection in highly susceptible or immunocompromised patients (Rutala and Weber, 1997). Biofilm may form in bulk water storage tanks and pipework and these should be examined at intervals and if necessary cleaned and/or chlorinated. When using covered supply tanks, checking and replacement of lids is also important. Heating water dechlorinates it and water standing in tanks or unused lengths of pipework or trapped around, tap washers may produce an increase in bacterial counts. Despite these problems tap water is very rarely an infection risk to the healthy person.

Water used to rinse away disinfectant residues from instruments and medical equipment should be of a suitable microbiological quality, i.e. autoclaved or filtered using a bacteria-retaining filter of 0.45 or 0.2 μm. This is particularly important for invasive items or those entering sterile body cavities.

Another problematic micro-organism found in hospital water supplies is *Legionella* (see also Chapters 2 and 3), which are ubiquitous in environmental waters and, on occasions, can be isolated from hospital water tanks, cooling towers, evaporator condensers, calorifiers and associated pipework. Growth is favoured by high levels of ferric salts, e.g. rust, and occurs between 20°C and 50°C. *Legionella* can multiply in the presence of free-living amoebae and if water is allowed to stagnate, and is then aerosolized, it can cause respiratory infections.

Infection control practitioners must adhere to national good practice guidelines, i.e. *The Control of Legionella in Health Care Premises* (NHS Estates, 1993b). Approved biocides must be used and the Director of Estates must ensure that the water storage tanks, calorifiers and cooling towers are regularly drained, cleaned and disinfected, and that a record of this is kept. This is particularly important following water system replacement or disturbance during upgrading work. The temperature of the supply at the outlets should be below 20°C or above 50°C. If this is achieved it will discourage the proliferation of *Legionella*. An improved design for cooling towers which avoids aerosol production is advised for new buildings.

Showers are also a small, but identifiable *Legionella* risk and *Legionella* grow on some rubber washers and seals. Dead legs in pipework should be avoided where possible and showers designed to eliminate static water. *Legionella* antagonistic seals should be used where possible.

Hydrotherapy pools

The structure of hydrotherapy pools, the use of water and intermittent and often extensive use by diverse groups including infected and severely immunocompromised patients, all produce potentially hazardous conditions (PHLS Working Party, 1994). Specific infections due to mycobacteria, adenoviruses, enteroviruses, amoebae and pseudomonas are well documented and so are poolside infections of the feet by epidermophytes.

The management of hydrotherapy pools should be placed in the hands of a senior physiotherapist with support from a microbiologist, engineer and the Infection Control Team. The pool manager should be responsible for cleaning, disinfection and maintenance and for keeping a record of activities in this respect. Advice on pool management may be found in the PHLS booklet on *Hygiene for Spa Pools* (1994).

The primary aim is to keep pools safe, pleasant to use and free of irritant substances and high numbers of potentially pathogenic micro-organisms. Bathers introduce skin squames, cosmetics, mucus, sebaceous and other secretions and often faeces and urine, to pool waters. These increase the likelihood of contamination and microbial proliferation. The frequent exchange of water, chlorination, pH adjustment and the use of filters all minimize the risk of significant contamination.

To reduce microbial contamination the water should be dosed with a chlorine-releasing agent, e.g. sodium hypochlorite or dichloroisocyanurate, to give a residual free-chlorine concentration in the range 1.5–3 ppm. A temporary 2–5-fold increase in levels may be necessary following faecal contamination or the growth of algae. Higher concentrations of 100–200 ppm are used for poolside surfaces and the irrigation of pumps, pipework and other pool-associated equipment. Regular monitoring of chlorine concentrations, water hardness, pH and turbidity are essential in good pool management.

Periodic sampling for bacteria is advised, although there is no absolute agreement on frequency. The report must give a total viable count of bacteria after incubation for 24 h at 37°C. If counts are in excess of 100 colony-forming units per ml, reference should be made to the presence or absence of *Pseudomonas* spp. coliforms and *Staph. aureus*. Further information on pool management may then be required or should there be any adverse health effect.

Single patient hydrotherapy and birthing baths, particularly those of the whirlpool or Jacuzzi type, are popular with patients but are notoriously difficult to decontaminate between patients as they have pumps which recirculate the water. These are difficult to drain, clean and disinfect. The non-recirculatory type of baths are preferred as they are easily drained by removing a plug and the walls and base can be cleaned and disinfected with a non-abrasive chlorine-releasing agent. If recirculatory systems are used, the pump unit and associated pipework must be accessible for cleaning and disinfection. Chlorine-releasing agents are often damaging to pump components in the long term. An effective, non-damaging disinfectant should be used between patients and at the start of each session. Advice on component compatibility with disinfectants should be sought from equipment manufacturers.

References

Ayliffe, G.A.J. (1974) The role of ventilation systems in the prevention of hospital infection. *J. Inst. Hosp. Eng.*, **48**(5), 6–8.

Ayliffe, G.A.J., Babb, J.R. and Collins, B.J. (1974a) Carpets in hospital wards. *Health Soc. Serv. J.*, Oct.

Ayliffe, G.A.J., Babb, J.R., Collins, B.J., *et al.* (1974b) *Pseudomonas aeruginosa* in hospital sinks. *Lancet*, **2**, 578–581.

Ayliffe, G.A.J., Babb, J.R. and Collins, B.J. (1976) Environmental hazards – real and imaginary. *Health Soc. Serv. J.*, (suppl.), June 26.

Ayliffe, G.A.J., Babb, J.R., Taylor, L. and Wise, R. (1979) A unit for source and protective isolation in a general hospital. *Br. Med. J.*, **2**, 461–465.

Ayliffe, G.A.J., Collins, B.J., Lowbury, E.J.L., *et al.* (1967) Ward floors and other surfaces as reservoirs of hospital infection. *J. Hyg. (Camb.)*, **65**, 515–535.

Collins, B.J. (1979) How to have carpeted luxury. *Health Soc. Serv. J.*, (suppl.), Sept. 28.

Collins, B.J. (1988) The hospital environment: how clean should it be? *J. Hosp. Infect.*, **11**, (Suppl. A), 53–56.

Lilly, H.A., Kidson, A. and Fujita, K. (1982) Investigation of hospital infection from a damaged mattress. *Burns*, **8**, 408–413.

Lowbury, E.J.L. and Ayliffe, G.A.J. (1982) Airborne infection in hospitals. *J. Hosp. Infect.*, **3**, 217–240.

Lowbury, E.J.L., Thom, B.T., Lilly, H.A., *et al.* (1970) Sources of infection with *Pseudomonas aeruginosa* in patients with tracheostomy. *J. Med. Microbiol.*, **3**(1), 39–56.

NHS Estates (1993a) *Ventilation in Healthcare Premises*, Health Technical Memorandum 2025, London, HMSO.

NHS Estates (1993b) *The Control of Legionellae in Healthcare Premises – A Code of Practice*, Health Technical Memorandum 2040, London, HMSO.

PHLS Working Party (1994) *Hygiene for Spa Pools*, Public Health Laboratory Service, 61 Colindale Avenue, London NW9 5DF.

Rutala, W.A. and Weber, D.J. (1997) Water as a reservoir of nosocomial pathogens. *Infect. Control Hosp. Epidemiol.*, **18**(9), 609–616.

9

Cleaning, disinfection or sterilization?

Cleaning, disinfection and sterilization are processes which remove or destroy micro-organisms. They are therefore used to prevent contact transmission on instruments, equipment, environmental surfaces and the skin. The method of decontamination chosen will depend largely on the nature of potential pathogens present and on the infection risk associated with the surface or device (Medical Devices Agency, 1993/96).

It is sometimes difficult to make a choice between different methods. Some, although highly effective, are expensive and more likely to damage the structure and function of the item or to keep it out of commission for long periods. There is little sense in selecting an elaborate process of sterilization if the organisms present are unlikely to cause infection or will reappear before the device is next used. To obtain a completely sterile environment would be prohibitively expensive and impractical as well as unnecessary. Even if achieved, it would not be maintained if people, the principal sources of micro-organisms, were present within the environment. There is little point in destroying micro-organisms if this is not associated with a reduction in infection risk or if an acceptable or low level of contamination cannot be maintained. Disinfecting a lavatory seat once a week could influence the risk of infection to the next user but not for subsequent users. A more logical approach is to identify the individual likely to contaminate the seat with pathogens and always disinfect after use by him/her. The following may assist the reader in making a logical choice as to which method of decontamination is most appropriate.

Choice of decontamination method

Decontamination is a process which reduces or destroys contaminants and thereby prevents micro-organisms or other unwanted material reaching a susceptible site in sufficient quantities to initiate infection or some other harmful response. The choice of decontamination method will depend on many factors in addition to infection risk, e.g. the nature of contamination, the time available for processing, the heat, pressure, moisture and chemical tolerance of the item, the availability of processing equipment and the quality of, and the risks associated with, the decontamination method.

Heat sterilization or disinfection methods are preferred, but if the item is heat sensitive, chemicals may have to be used. It is essential that the process selected is effective against patient-associated micro-organisms and opportunistic pathogens likely to be present in the environment. The use of validated, automated processes are preferred for high- or intermediate-risk items such as those which are invasive or in contact with infectious material. These are usually safe and reliable, provided that the equipment is suitably monitored and maintained and that staff wear appropriate protective clothing. Invasive items should be packed prior to sterilization to prevent environmental contamination after processing.

Sterilization

This is a process which destroys or removes all living micro-organisms including bacterial spores. It renders medical devices free from viable micro-organisms and is recommended for all items penetrating intact skin or mucous membranes or entering vascular systems or sterile body cavities. Items sterilized are usually packaged or contained to protect them from recontamination while being stored for reuse.

Disinfection

This is a process which reduces the number of viable micro-organisms but which may not inactivate some bacterial spores. Disinfection may not necessarily achieve the same reduction in microbial contamination levels as sterilization and is usually associated with items which are not intentionally invasive but are in contact with mucous membranes, infectious material, blood and other body fluids. Disinfection is also a process widely used in sterile service departments and other decontamination centres to ensure that dirty returned surgical instruments and medical equipment are safe for staff to handle prior to inspection, repair and processing for reuse. The process may also be used for invasive items if no practical means of sterilization is available.

Cleaning

Cleaning physically removes micro-organisms and the organic material on which they thrive. It does not necessarily destroy micro-organisms but removes them and other contaminants, e.g. chemical residues, degradation products, soil, dust, pyrogens, radioactive and any other material which would otherwise adversely affect the performance of the device. Cleaning is an essential prerequisite to disinfection and sterilization and, if not effectively carried out, may influence the performance of the sterilant or disinfectant.

A classification of infection risk associated with the decontamination of medical devices and surfaces is given in Table 9.1. Methods of decontamination are indicated, together with examples of the items and surfaces processed.

Table 9.1   Classification of items and surfaces in relation to risk

Risk category	Method of decontamination	Process options	Examples of items/ surfaces
High risk In contact with a break in the skin or mucous membrane. Entry into sterile cavities or vascular systems	Cleaning and sterilization	*Heat tolerant* Autoclave, hot air oven *Heat sensitive* Single use, ethylene oxide, low-temperature steam and formaldehyde, sporicidal disinfectants, e.g. glutaraldehyde, peracetic acid	Surgical instruments, invasive endoscopes, e.g. laparoscopes, cardiac catheters, implants, infusions, injections, needles, syringes, swabs, surgical dressings, sutures
Intermediate risk In contact with intact mucous membranes, body fluids or other potentially infectious material	Cleaning and disinfection (or sterilization)	All the above and *Heat tolerant* Boiling, pasteurization, low temperature steam, washer disinfectors *Heat sensitive* Disinfectants	Respiratory and anaesthetic equipment, non-invasive endoscopes, e.g. gastroscopes, thermometers, vaginal speculae, body fluid spills, dirty instruments prior to reprocessing, bed pans and urine bottles
Low risk In contact with intact healthy skin	Cleaning usually adequate (disinfection if known infection risk)	All the above and manual cleaning with soap or detergent, automated cleaning/ disinfection, disinfectants	Trolley tops, operating table, wash-bowls, lavatory seats, baths, wash hand basins, bedding, patient supports
Minimal risk Remote, not in direct contact with patients	Cleaning alone	Manual or automated cleaning, damp dusting, wet mopping, dust attractant mops, vacuum cleaners	Floors, walls, furniture, ceilings, drains

Transmissible degenerative (spongiform) encephalopathies

At this time, little is known about the causes, transmission, diagnosis, prevention and cure of patients with transmissible spongiform encephalopathies, which include Creutzfeldt–Jakob disease (CJD), scrapie and bovine spongiform encephalopathy (BSE). It should not be assumed that the methods described in subsequent chapters of this book are necessarily effective against such agents. Few of the current methods of sterilization and disinfection are effective in inactivating these agents (Taylor, 1992, see p. 166).

Single use devices

Some items, particularly those which are invasive, constructed of heat-sensitive components or are difficult to clean, are manufactured and labelled as single use. These are packaged and sterilized by the manufacturer who takes responsibility for the quality and safety of the item, provided that it is used once only and is not reprocessed. This option is preferred by many users as it offers a safer and more convenient alternative to internal processing, particularly if toxic and irritant chemicals are used. However, single use may prove prohibitively expensive, particularly in developing countries and those with limited financial and reprocessing resources.

It is clearly in the manufacturers' interest to label items as single use because there would be little commercial incentive to produce reprocessable items if hospitals keep buying single use ones. If a single use device is reprocessed the manufacturer is no longer responsible for subsequent deficiencies. Although this would seem reasonable, the processors are unwilling to expose themselves to possible litigation, especially as a number of warnings to this effect have been sent out by the manufacturers and some national authorities. In spite of this, reuse of single use items is widespread throughout the world and there would appear to be little or no evidence of infection or damage to patients. A possible solution to this dilemma is that the health care establishment concerned should set up a Device Assessment Group. This would comprise of an infection control doctor and nurse, sterile service manager (or processor) and a risk assessor. The person wishing to reuse the single use device should present the case to the group, providing the reason for the request and other relevant information, e.g. cost, preference for particular item, integration with existing systems, etc. If, having considered the safety and cost effectiveness associated with reuse, a decision is made to reuse, a report should be issued to the chief executive or senior administrator. A corporate decision can then be made on reuse and the hospital or health care establishment must then become legally responsible for the item.

Advice from the Department of Health in the UK (Medical Devices Agency, 1995) states that medical devices labelled as single use should not be processed and reused unless the reprocessor:

- is able to apply and achieve the stringent technical requirements necessary to ensure the integrity and safety of each reprocessed item
- can produce documentary proof and evidence of successful validation of the reprocessing operation. These studies are for the purpose of confirming that the reprocessing method chosen produces a safe and cost effective product, fit for the intended purpose
- has a system for retaining full reprocessing batch records, for subsequent retrieval in the event of a device failure or patient injury.

Manufacturers should be encouraged to produce information on suitable decontamination processes and should give the users the opportunity to purchase either reusable or single use items. The rapidly expanding use of single use devices is a major factor in the increase of clinical waste. From an ecological standpoint, single use items should be replaced with reusable items wherever possible.

Decontamination policies

It is the responsibility of the Infection Control Committee (ICC) to produce a decontamination policy. The formulation and implementation of this policy is the responsibility of the Infection Control Team (ICT). Should a problem occur with decontamination, the processor, e.g. Sterile Services Manager, nurse or technician, should liaise initially with the ICT who will either resolve the problem or refer it back to the ICC.

It is strongly advised that information on suitable methods of cleaning, disinfection and sterilization are sought before formulating local policy. National guidelines should be used wherever possible. Sources of information in the UK include:

- The Department of Health, Medical Devices Agency, NHS estates
- Professional societies, e.g. Institute of Sterile Services Management, Central Sterilizing Club, Hospital Infection Society, Infection Control Nurses' Association and Institute of Healthcare Engineering and Estate Management
- Reference centres and research establishments, e.g. Central Public Health Laboratory, Hospital Infection Research Laboratory
- Books, working party reports and journals (see bibliography)
- British, European and International Standards, e.g. BSI, CEN, ISO
- Manufacturers, e.g. of instruments, medical equipment, sterilizers, washer disinfectors, disinfectants, etc.

The following factors should be considered before deciding upon a suitable decontamination process:

- Is the item intended for reuse? – establish that it is not described as single use
- For what purpose is the device used? – is it invasive, in contact with mucous membranes, skin, body fluids or other potentially infectious material?
- How do the manufacturers describe it should be cleaned, disinfected or sterilized?
- Can it be disassembled to facilitate cleaning?
- Is decontamination required at the point of use?
- Will it withstand an automated cleansing process?
- Do you have an appropriate sterilization or disinfection facility?
- Can it be wrapped to protect it from recontamination prior to use?
- How many times can it be reprocessed?
- Does reprocessing constitute a hazard to patients and staff? If so, are Control of Substances Hazardous to Health (COSHH) hazard data, personal protective and monitoring equipment available?

A review of process options for cleaning, disinfection and sterilization can be found in Chapters 10 (cleaning), 11 (disinfection) and 12 (sterilization). Wherever possible, reusable items should be manufactured which are accessible for cleaning and that are disinfected or sterilized using heat.

References

Medical Devices Agency (1993/96) *Sterilization, Disinfection and Cleaning of Medical Equipment: Guidance on Decontamination Part 1: Principles; Part 2: Protocols; and Part 3: Procedures* (in preparation), Microbiology Advisory Committee to the Department of Health, London, HMSO.

Medical Devices Agency (1995) *The Reuse of Medical Devices Supplied for Single Use Only*, MDA Device Bulletin 9501, London, Department of Health.

Taylor, D.M. (1992) Inactivation of unconventional agents of the transmissible degenerative encephalopathies. In *Principles and Practice of Disinfection, Preservation and Sterilization*, 2nd edn. (A.D. Russell, W.B. Hugo and G.A.J. Ayliffe, eds), Oxford, Blackwell Publications, pp.171–179.

10

Cleaning

Regular and efficient cleaning is necessary to maintain the appearance, structure and function of health care buildings and their contents. It is also required to control the microbial population and to prevent odour and the transfer of potentially infectious material (Collins, 1988). Cleaning alone may be sufficient for items and surfaces which are remote from the patient or that are in contact with normal healthy skin (see Chapter 9), but it is also a prerequisite to satisfactory disinfection or sterilization.

Cleaning is a process intended to remove contamination and this includes any harmful or undesirable substance. In clinical situations this is likely to be excretions, secretions and micro-organisms, but may also include dust, grease and the residual products of sterilization and disinfection. If contaminants are not removed they may have an adverse effect on the patient or the function of the surface or device.

Cleaning removes micro-organisms and the organic material on which they thrive. It also removes substances which would otherwise protect pathogenic micro-organisms during sterilization or disinfection, particularly if chemical agents are used (Ayliffe et al., 1993). Cleaning should be achieved without shortening the life or interfering with the function of the device. After cleaning, surfaces should have fewer organisms present and will be of lower infection risk. Cleaning with dirty, moist mops and wipes is ineffective and may add to the number of micro-organisms present. The sources of 'soil' and micro-organisms are many and include skin squames and particles deposited from the air and transferred by contact with people, their clothing and inanimate objects.

Cleaning to the required standards requires specialized training and the use of effective procedures, equipment and materials.

Environment: structure and function

A clean environment in hospitals and other health care buildings is essential, as failure to meet expected standards can seriously reduce patients' confidence in the ability of the hospital to provide safe and effective medical care. The accumulation of dirt may mask important identification marks, warnings or instructions. It may also corrode or damage surfaces, block lumens and impair the flow of liquids, gases or electric current in medical equipment.

Also, accumulations of rubbish, body fluids and spilt food encourages the presence of insects, rodents and other pests. A warm environment, dirt and moisture provide ideal conditions for the proliferation of bacteria. If the risk of infection transmission is to be minimized, drying is also an essential part of the cleaning process.

Cleaning procedures

Cleaning should remove and not redistribute soil, body fluids and micro-organisms. The method of removal requires careful consideration. Cleaning should not increase the number of micro-organisms in the surrounding environment and any redispersal should be kept to a minimum (Ayliffe *et al.*, 1966). If a technique is used which disperses organisms into the air and it cannot be avoided, cleaning should not be carried out in the immediate vicinity of patients with exposed wounds or other susceptible sites unless these can be covered. Alternatively the area should be vacated and sufficient time left to allow the dispersed organisms to settle before the room is reoccupied.

Some environmental sites, e.g. drains, lavatory pans, urinals and sink outlets, are naturally heavily contaminated with Gram-negative bacteria and cleaning will only have a very temporary influence on their numbers. Although these areas must be kept clean, it is often more sensible to regard them as contaminated and to take any necessary precautions to prevent transmission rather than to adopt expensive and often ineffective measures and then ignore the risk. However, the risks of infection from drains, toilets, sinks, etc., is generally small (see Chapter 8).

Methods of cleaning environmental surfaces

Two basic methods of cleaning are used, i.e. dry and wet (Ayliffe *et al.*, 1967). If a dry method is used, dispersal of bacteria-carrying particles into the air is the main infection risk. The organisms primarily involved are Gram-positive cocci from the skin. *Staph. aureus* is the main pathogen and is responsible for approximately one-third of postoperative wound infections. Anaerobic spore-bearing bacilli, such as *Clostridium perfringens* or *Cl. tetani*, may be present in small numbers. These organisms will only cause infection if introduced into deep, oxygen-deficient tissues and their presence in small numbers in the environment is no cause for concern. Dry methods rely on mechanical action to loosen and remove soil. They do not remove stains and are unsuitable for wet or greasy surfaces. Wet cleaning methods are more suitable for dirty, hard surfaces and spillage. These do not raise dust and rarely increase airborne infection risk.

Dry methods

Sweeping
Brooms tend to redisperse bacteria-laden particles into the air, even when used with care. This may increase the airborne bacteria-carrying particle

Table 10.1   Changes in airborne bacterial counts associated with different methods of cleaning floors*

Cleaning method used	Change in the numbers of bacteria carrying particles in the air†
1. Sweeping with broom	700% increase
2. Vacuum cleaning	20% decrease
3. Dust-attracting floor mop	30% increase
4. Wet scrubbing machine	3% increase

* Studies carried out at the Hospital Infection Research Laboratory, City Hospital, Birmingham.† The effect may vary with the type of equipment used, the area being cleaned and the method of use.

count as much as 10-fold (Table 10.1). Dispersed dust will then resettle. Sweeping is, therefore, potentially hazardous and inefficient and should be avoided in clinical and food preparation areas.

Dust attractant mops
Mops which are specially treated or manufactured to attract and retain dust particles, i.e. sticky or static, cause much smaller increases in airborne counts (Table 10.1) and remove more dust from surfaces than brooms (Babb *et al.*, 1963; Collins *et al.*, 1972). Tests indicate that dry mops require washing or reprocessing after about 2 days use, although this will depend on the location of use and soiling. Their dust-holding properties may be extended to 4 or 5 days if the head is vacuumed after each use. The method of use is important if dispersal is to be avoided; the head of the mop should be kept flat and in close contact with the floor and not tilted or lifted at the end of each stroke. Mops of this type, with a disposable head, are available but are more expensive.

Vacuum cleaning
Vacuum cleaners are now widely used in hospitals for carpeted areas. A well-designed vacuum cleaner should not increase airborne counts, provided that the exhausted air is passed through a bacteria-retaining filter or bag (Table 10.1). The expelled air from the cleaners should be diffused and directed away from the floor so that it does not blow the dust from uncleaned surfaces.

Dusting
Dry dusting, particularly if high, may dislodge or disperse dust and micro-organisms onto the patient. Damp dusting is preferable, although dry dusting can be carried out with a vacuum head or a dust-attractant mop. If there is a danger of dispersing dust, all open wounds should be kept covered for at least 30 min after dusting has ceased.

Wet methods

Scrubbing and mopping
Detergents, solvents and descalers may be used to suspend, dissolve and remove adherent soil. Dispersal of micro-organisms into the air is less likely

during wet cleaning than dry cleaning (Table 10.1). However, cleaning solutions soon become contaminated and bacteria may grow in them. Splashes or aerosols produced by wet cleaning methods are therefore likely to be contaminated with potential pathogens such as Gram-negative bacilli. Used cleaning solutions should be disposed of promptly and safely. Bacteria removed from the surface are transferred to the mop bucket and this water should be changed frequently or a two-bucket system (fresh and soiled) used. It is usually necessary, particularly in operating theatres, to rinse surfaces after cleaning, as detergents and soap residues will build up on the surface when the fluid dries out. This will increase the rate of soil accumulation, interfere with the antistatic properties of theatre floors and may attack finishes. The residual film may also be slippery and interfere with subsequent treatments by preventing bonding with the surface.

Moist surfaces encourage bacterial growth and should be regarded as a potential infection hazard. After cleaning, food preparation and clinical work surfaces should not be used until they are completely dry. If excessive amounts of detergent are used, and a wet vacuum machine is used to remove residual cleaning solution, foam may prevent the shut-off valve from functioning correctly and a bacterial aerosol may be produced from the exhaust. This is a potential infection hazard. Vacuum exhaust systems are also used on carpets following hot water or steam cleaning, as rapid drying is important in reducing contamination and suppressing unpleasant odours.

Routine cleaning should be carried out as part of an agreed policy, with detailed schedules. Hospital policy should be given preference where it conflicts with cleaning equipment and material manufacturers' instructions, but it is always a good idea to read the instructions first and clarify any discrepancies with policy.

Washer disinfectors

Automated systems are the preferred method of cleaning and disinfecting a wide range of items including surgical instruments, endoscopes, holloware, anaesthetic equipment, bedpans, urinals, crockery, cutlery and catering equipment (Babb, 1993; Medical Devices Agency, 1993/96). A full account of the merits and testing of this type of equipment is given in Chapter 11. It is important to show that these machines clean items thoroughly. This may be done by regularly checking the cleanliness of processed items or by applying an artificial soil to specific testpieces and assessing the effectiveness of soil removal (British Standards Institution, 1993). Failures to clean are usually caused by: too high an initial wash temperature (which causes protein to coagulate), blocked jets or drains, the use of an unsuitable detergent or improper loading which results in a shadowing effect.

Outline policy for good manual cleaning practice

1. Wearing suitable protective clothing, i.e. apron and gloves, prepare a fresh cleaning solution appropriately diluted for each task. Make up only the quantity required in a clean, dry container. Freshly drawn tap

water is usually suitable, but very hard water will precipitate soaps and neutralize some disinfectants. Hand-hot water removes oils and fats and cleans better than cold, but at very high temperatures protein, e.g. milk and blood, coagulates and will be more difficult to remove.

2. Apply the cleaning solution evenly to all the surfaces. If a brush, mop or wipe is used it should be clean and preferably dry before use.

3. Do not put more fluid than necessary onto a surface. This avoids waste, seepage into cracks, fabric shrinkage and difficulties with subsequent removal.

4. Change the solution frequently to prevent a build-up of soil or micro-organisms which would recontaminate the surface.

5. Allow sufficient time for cleaning solutions to penetrate the soil on the surface, but remember that strong acid and alkaline cleaning agents can damage surfaces if left for too long.

6. Rinse off cleaning solutions when practical.

7. Dispose of cleaning solution promptly in a sluice or sink in the dirty utility area. Do not discard into wash hand basins.

8. Expel any fluid trapped in lumens and dry the surface as thoroughly as possible.

9. Remove cleaning equipment from clinical or food preparation areas as soon as possible. Make sure it is cleaned, dried and stored in a designated place. If the equipment is faulty it should be reported promptly to a supervisor and either repaired or replaced.

10. Remove gloves and protective clothing and wash hands before carrying out any other duties.

Hospital cleaning is a specialized task which requires well-supervised, trained staff who will keep to the detailed schedules produced by the Hotel Services Manager in consultation with the departmental manager and members of the Infection Control Team. Alternative cleaning methods or materials should not be used unless authorized. Some cleaning products are incompatible and should only be mixed if this is approved by the manufacturer. Soaps or detergents often reduce the effectiveness of disinfectants and some products may react in a dangerous manner, e.g. soap neutralizes quarternary ammonium compounds and acid cleaners react violently with chlorine-releasing agents to produce chlorine, a poisonous gas. Not all the cleaning techniques used in hospitals have been properly planned, co-ordinated and adequately researched. It is sensible to investigate cleaning methods which are used and for which the choice does not appear to be scientifically based. It is the responsibility of infection control staff to liaise with other disciplines in evaluating new cleaning procedures in relation to infection risk.

Cleaning of isolation cubicles and other special or high-risk areas

Specialized techniques, which are not justified in other areas, may be required for operating theatres, intensive care units and isolation rooms occupied by infected or highly susceptible patients. Detailed schedules for cleaning these areas should be produced in consultation with the Hotel Services Manager, senior nursing staff and members of the ICT. The cleaning techniques selected may vary with location and infection risk. Disinfectants are not usually necessary, but firm decisions should be made as to whether or not they are required.

The following objectives should be considered when formulating a cleaning policy:

1. Microbial contamination from an infected patient should be contained within that room, cubicle or locality.
2. The patient should be protected from additional infection risk.
3. Anyone with access to that environment should be aware of the measures required to prevent the spread of infection.
4. After use by an infected patient the environment should be made safe for any future occupancy or use and it should be apparent that this has been done.

Some of the main considerations when formulating a cleaning policy for isolation cubicles are outlined below:

1. The sister in charge of the ward should notify the domestic supervisor as soon as possible that special cleaning is required. The domestic supervisor should then ensure that:

    (a) the correct procedure is known and understood by the domestic staff responsible and that suitable protective clothing and materials are available
    (b) the domestic staff are sufficiently aware of any risks to themselves or others, and are adequately protected; for example, if the patient has open pulmonary tuberculosis, only tuberculin-positive staff are used
    (c) cubicles are cleaned in the right order, i.e. the cubicles used for the isolation of highly susceptible patients should be cleaned before those of infected patients and staff should not re-enter that cubicle until the cleaning of cubicles for infected patients is complete and suitable measures to prevent transfer have been taken.

2. Equipment should be reserved for use in the specified area only, and clearly marked for that purpose; it must be stored in this area, or in a clearly designated place outside it. Where this is not possible, equipment must be adequately decontaminated immediately after each use. The use of automated cleaning equipment should be avoided if possible in isolation rooms for infected patients but, if used, a separate brush or head should be reserved for use in that area and this should be decontaminated, preferably by thermal disinfection or autoclaving, before use elsewhere. The outside of the machine should be wiped after use with a suitable disinfectant, e.g. a chlorine-releasing agent or clear soluble phenolic. Scrubbing machines with tanks are particularly difficult to decontaminate and their use should be avoided in high-risk areas. Use of disposable wipes which can be discarded inside the isolation cubicle prevents their accidental reuse in other areas.

Cleaning equipment should be kept to a minimum. The following will usually suffice:

- a plastic bag for the disposal of domestic (black) or clinical waste (yellow)
- a bowl for damp dusting, preferably kept dry and stored within the cubicle
- an appropriate disinfectant solution if required
- a mop and bucket designated for use in that area only
- disposable paper wipes.

Procedure

1. Collect all the equipment required for cleaning.
2. Enter the cubicle, wash hands, put on disposable apron and gloves.
3. Pick up any large items of rubbish and discard into an appropriate waste bag. Sweeping is unacceptable. A vacuum cleaner is rarely necessary unless a carpet is fitted. If used, a dedicated machine is preferred.
4. Clean the floor with a damp mop.
5. Make up a solution of disinfectant (if required) in a bowl. Use disposable wipes moistened in the solution to clean surfaces. Clean structural items first, including the door handles. Clean furnishings, starting with the locker and finishing with the waste bin and sink. Discard remaining cleaning solution in the bucket, wipe the bowl and return to the storage area in the cubicle.
6. Remove gloves and plastic apron and, if single use, discard into plastic bag; seal bag; wash and dry the hands.
7. Leave the cubicle, taking with you the sealed rubbish bag and any item of equipment not stored in the cubicle. Buckets should be emptied, dried and returned to the storage area. Occasionally it is specified that the cleaning water is disposed of inside the cubicle, although this is often impractical. This means that grossly contaminated fluids are tipped into a hand-basin or toilet, possibly splashing the recently cleaned surface. If this is likely to occur, reserve some cleaning solution to reclean the splashed surfaces. If dirty cleaning fluid is removed from the cubicle, it should be taken immediately to the dirty utility room, discarded, the bucket cleaned and the hands washed.

When an infected patient is removed from an isolation cubicle, a notice such as 'DO NOT USE', should be put on the door. The notice should only be removed by a senior nurse after checking that all necessary decontamination measures have taken place, surfaces are dry and that the cubicle is safe to reoccupy.

Contract cleaning

It is now common practice to contract out domestic, catering, portering and laundry services. All staff working in clinical and food preparation areas from these disciplines must have a sound knowledge of infection control and food hygiene procedures relevant to their work area, and appropriate training must therefore be given. This is likely to be expensive and provision should be made for this when negotiating contracts. Where a requirement exists for contractual workers to have regular health checks, or to be immunized against specific infections, e.g. tetanus, rubella, polio, HBV or tuberculosis, this must also be considered.

The equipment, materials and cleaning methods used by contractors should conform with existing hospital policy. Supervision of the contract to ensure compliance with infection control and health and safety policies is vital. Regular audits are a way of doing this, but those responsible for carrying out such a task, e.g. ICNs, must be consulted when drawing up the contract. Administrative problems are likely to occur if contractors are unaware of health and safety and infection control policies and the nature and frequency of audits.

Effective monitoring of cleaning schedules requires a considerable amount of time, specialized skills and sometimes laboratory services. Those infection control practitioners who are expected to carry out this task may not have the appropriate resources available. Some flexibility should exist within contracts to allow for changes or the implementation of additional procedures should this be necessary during outbreaks.

References

Ayliffe, G.A.J., Collins, B.J. and Lowbury, E.J.L. (1966) Cleaning and disinfection of hospital floors. *Br. Med. J.*, **2**, 442–445.

Ayliffe, G.A.J, Collins, B.J., Lowbury, E.J.L., *et al.* (1967) Ward floors and other surfaces as reservoirs of hospital infection. *J. Hyg. (Lond.)*, **65**, 515–535.

Ayliffe, G.A.J., Coates, D. and Hoffman, P.N. (1993) *Chemical Disinfection in Hospitals*, London, Public Health Laboratory Services.

Babb, J.R. (1993) Methods of cleaning and disinfection. *Central Sterilization, Central Service*, official publication of European Society of Hospital Sterile Supply, **4**, 227–237.

Babb, J.R., Lilly, H.A. and Lowbury, E.J.L. (1963) Cleaning of hospital floors with oiled mops. *J. Hyg. (Camb.)*, **61**, 393.

British Standards Institution (1993) *Washer Disinfectors for Medical Purposes*, British Standard 2745 Parts 1–3, London, British Standards Institution.

Collins, B.J. (1988) The hospital environment: how clean should it be? *J. Hosp. Inf.*, **11** (suppl. A), 53–56.

Collins, B.J., Wilkins, M. and Ayliffe, G. (1972) Dry cleaning of hospital floors. *Br. Hosp. J. Social Service Rev.*, 9 December.

Medical Devices Agency (1993/96) *Sterilization, Disinfection and Cleaning of Medical Equipment: Guidance on Decontamination. Part 1: Principles; part 2: Protocols; and part 3: Procedures* (in preparation), London, HMSO.

11

Disinfection

Disinfection is a process used to reduce the number of viable micro-organisms on a surface or in a load, but which may not necessarily inactivate some viruses and bacterial spores. Disinfection may not achieve the same reduction in microbial contamination levels as sterilization (Medical Devices Agency, 1993/96, 1996) and is usually associated with those items that are not intentionally invasive, but are in contact with mucous membranes, body fluids and other potentially infectious material. It may also be used for invasive items, or those in contact with a breach in the skin or mucous membranes, if no practical means of sterilization is available.

It is difficult to see why certain viruses are included as a possible exception. Viruses are more susceptible to disinfectants than most mycobacteria, and it may be worth while considering different levels of disinfection, e.g. high-level disinfection would include effectiveness against *Mycobacterium tuberculosis*. A revision of the definition might be worth while. A modification of Dr J.C. Kelsey's proposal to the original Committee on Standardisation of Disinfection in Europe is worth considering, i.e.: Disinfection is the selective elimination of certain undesirable micro-organisms to an extent that it is considered safe by a competent authority for a particular purpose.

Most equipment-associated infection is due to inadequate cleaning and disinfection and not to a failure in sterilization practices (Ayliffe, 1988). The method of disinfection chosen should relate to the risks associated with the procedures undertaken (see Chapter 9), the heat, pressure and chemical tolerances of the item and the time available for processing. Heat disinfection is preferred, but if the item is heat sensitive, or the treatment is impractical, disinfectants may have to be used. It is important that the method of disinfection is effective against patient-associated micro-organisms and opportunistic pathogens present in the environment. The most important stage of any decontamination procedure is thorough cleaning and this should accompany or precede all disinfection procedures (Babb, 1993b).

Disinfection is also a process whereby staff working in sterile services departments and elsewhere ensure that dirty returned surgical instruments and medical equipment are free from infection risk and safe to handle prior to processing for reuse. A summary of the various options for disinfection are shown in Table 11.1.

Thermal disinfection

Exposure to hot water or steam is the most effective, and usually the safest and least expensive, method of disinfection. Items normally decontaminated

Table 11.1   Disinfection: process options

Heat: Bedpans, urine bottles, linen, anaesthetic equipment, used instruments, suction bottles, ventilator circuits

Instrument boiler	100°C	5–10 min
Sub-atmospheric steam	73–80°C	10 min
Washer disinfectors	65°C	10 min
	71°C	3 min
	80°C	1 min
	90°C	1 s

Chemical: Spillage, heat-sensitive instruments and equipment

Formaldehyde vapour	Respiratory equipment, suction pumps, ventilators, laboratory safety cabinets, incubators
2% glutaraldehyde	Heat-sensitive instruments, e.g. some rigid and all flexible endoscopes
70% alcohol	Instruments, thermometers, trolley tops, medical equipment
Chlorine-releasing agents (125–10,000 ppm av Cl_2)	Blood/body fluid spillage, respiratory, dialysis and catering equipment, baby feed bottles
Clear soluble phenolics	Spillage, some instruments and holloware

in this way include hospital linen, bedpans, urinals, crockery, cutlery, suction bottles, surgical instruments and respiratory equipment. Process temperatures vary between 65°C and 100°C and usually the higher the temperature the shorter the processing time. Automated washer disinfectors (Figures 11.1) are preferred and the cycle parameters chosen will depend on the thermal tolerance of the item, the thoroughness of the cleansing process and the nature of contamination (British Standards Institution 1993 NHS

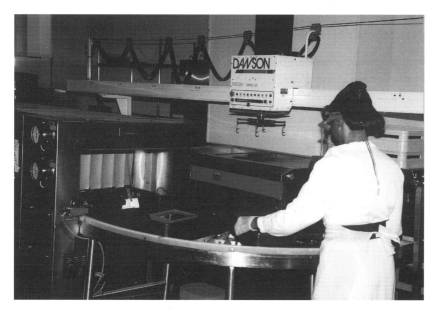

Figure 11.1   A thermal washer disinfector for used surgical instruments and holloware in a sterile services department

Estates HTM 2030 1995). In the UK linen, which is fairly heat sensitive, is processed at 65°C for 10 min or 71°C for 3 min (Barrie, 1994), whereas instruments that tolerate higher temperatures are processed in a washer disinfector which reaches 80–90°C for much shorter periods. Alternatively, if cleansing is not part of the automated process, boiling water is utilized, but for longer periods.

Boilers are still widely used in the community for precleaned instruments which are non-invasive, e.g. tongue depressors, vaginal speculae and proctoscopes, but their use has been discouraged because of the risk of scalds, removing items before they have reached disinfection temperatures or because of the recontamination risk, particularly if instruments are left to soak in water at room temperature for long periods. If used correctly so that clean items are immersed in boiling water which is allowed to reach 98–100°C and maintained for at least 5 min, they can disinfect reliably, but it is unlikely that the market for boilers will expand as there are now several comparatively inexpensive benchtop autoclaves which are quick, safe and will sterilize. These can be used for invasive and non-invasive items, especially by those remote from a sterile services department.

Sub-atmospheric steam at approximately 73°C is used in some hospitals for the disinfection of wrapped items such as ventilator circuits, face masks, ET tubes, airways and rigid endoscopes, in the latter case with or without formaldehyde (Medical Devices Agency, 1993/96, 1996). Machines are, however, expensive and items have to be thoroughly cleaned and dried first. In the UK preference is now shown for using washer disinfectors for respiratory equipment which clean, disinfect and dry during a single automated process. Items can then be packaged and stamped 'disinfected for reuse'.

Boiling water, or processing in a washer disinfector at temperatures between 65°C and 100°C, will destroy HIV, *Myco. tuberculosis* and most other non-sporing bacteria and viruses likely to pose a hazard to patients and staff. Although some doubt has been cast on the thermal tolerance of HBV at temperatures below 98°C, this is unlikely to survive, provided that thorough cleaning is a component of the decontamination process.

Washer disinfectors: monitoring performance

The performance of thermal washer disinfectors can be ascertained by monitoring the temperature of processed items and by checking soil removal. Thermocouples and a chart recorder can be attached to processed items to ensure that the specified time and temperature parameters are met or, if this is not practical, biological indicators may be used. Some strains of *Enterococcus faecalis* are particularly heat-resistant vegetative bacteria and an overnight broth culture, contained in a capillary or microcentrifuge tube, can be attached to the load (i.e. item of greatest mass), processed and cultured. No growth or at least a 5 $\log_{10}$ reduction (99.999%) will indicate that thermal disinfection has been achieved.

A range of soils which contain blood, egg yolk, hog mucin, wallpaper adhesive, dye and other ingredients have been devised for checking the cleaning performance of a wide range of washer disinfectors (British

Standards Institution, 1993). These are intended to mimic the behaviour of natural soil, but are safer, more standardized and acceptable than the real thing. Soil may be applied to a test load, e.g. set of surgical instruments, human waste receptacles or holloware. It is recommended that thermocouple and soil removal tests are carried out on commissioning, after machine maintenance or programme changes and at periodic intervals.

Tests have shown that cabinet and tunnel jet wash systems and ultrasonic washer disinfectors are highly effective in removing soil and micro-organisms, provided that dirty instruments are not subjected to heat before processing. In many hospitals, hazardous items are autoclaved or disinfected using low-temperature steam to make them safe for handling. This will bake or coagulate body fluids onto the instruments making subsequent removal difficult (Babb and Lynam, 1993). To ensure that blood and body fluids are removed before thermal disinfection, items should be subjected to a cool wash, i.e. below 35°C, to prevent protein coagulation. Higher temperatures are required to remove oils and fats and to disinfect the items.

Ultrasonic washer disinfectors are more efficient in cleaning the external surfaces of intricate items, particularly where blood and body fluids have dried onto surfaces, but they are not recommended for the telescopes of rigid endoscopes. Lumened devices require irrigation either by hand, using a high-pressure water jet, or by fluids pumped through the channels as part of an automated process. It is important that lumened items are flushed with cool water before subjecting them to heat which would coagulate protein and block the channel.

If hot water or steam is used to process unpacked items, they should be dried to prevent the proliferation of Gram-negative bacilli and other opportunistic pathogens acquired from the environment during storage.

Chemical disinfection

Formaldehyde cabinets

Formaldehyde vapour is occasionally used to disinfect rooms, laboratory safety cabinets and bulky items of medical equipment (Ayliffe *et al.*, 1992b). It is a slow sporicide and is only effective on clean, exposed surfaces. It is extremely irritant to the eyes, skin and respiratory tract and should not therefore be used unless it can be effectively contained and safely extracted and discharged. Most ventilators and suction pumps which were formerly disinfected with formaldehyde or hydrogen peroxide are now protected by bacteria-retaining filters, and environmental surfaces and small items can be more safely disinfected by exposure to hot water, steam or disinfectants.

Formaldehyde cabinets are available (Babb *et al.*, 1992) which preheat items to 36–40°C under controlled humitidy. Methanolized formalin is heated to generate formaldehyde vapour which is then circulated through the chamber and accessible parts of the load. Disinfection usually takes 3–8 h. Residual formaldehyde is neutralized with ammonia and the chamber and its contents finally flushed with air. Disinfection of ventilators and suction pumps is only achieved if formaldehyde is pumped throughout the circuits.

Disinfectants

A disinfectant is a chemical compound which destroys micro-organisms. Some disinfectants are non-toxic and can safely be applied to the skin or living tissues. These are called antiseptics. Others are capable of destroying spores and are referred to as sterilants. The use of these does not have the same degree of assurance as that achieved by physical methods such as autoclaving because items cannot be packaged to prevent recontamination before use and rinsing is necessary to remove toxic residues.

Disinfectants may be used to destroy potentially pathogenic organisms. Most are capable of destroying vegetative bacteria, fungi and viruses and are often the only means of processing heat-sensitive instruments and equipment outside a well-equipped hospital sterile services department.

Disinfectant policy

The Infection Control Team and Committee are those normally responsible for producing and implementing a disinfectant policy (Ayliffe *et al.*, 1993; Coates and Hutchinson, 1994). They may recruit the specialist services of a microbiologist, Safety Officer and pharmacist. The ICT may be sufficiently experienced to produce their own policy or may adopt the recommendations of the Department of Health, professional societies, reference centres or other specialist groups.

Factors taken into account when formulating a policy include: range of antimicrobial activity, surface compatibility, user friendliness, stability and cost (Babb, 1996). Micro-organisms vary in their susceptibility to disinfectants: Gram-positive bacteria are usually very susceptible, Gram-negative species less susceptible, mycobacteria are relatively resistant and spores highly resistant. Viruses vary according to their structure. Enveloped (lipid) viruses, such as herpes simplex and HIV are more sensitive than non-enveloped viruses, but on the whole these are more susceptible than mycobacteria and spores.

There is no ideal disinfectant. The relative merits of each product should be assessed and those which meet the greatest number of requirements selected. The properties of several widely used instrument and environmental disinfectants are shown Table 11.2. The most efficacious agents are often those which damage surfaces or that are toxic and sensitizing. New Health and Safety legislation in the UK, i.e. Control of Substances Hazardous to Health Regulations (COSHH), requires disinfectant users to carry out a careful assessment of the consequences of using hazardous substances. Some of the most effective disinfectants, e.g. glutaraldehyde and the chlorine-releasing agents, are irritant to the skin, eyes and respiratory tract. User-friendly alternatives are available, but the majority are less effective and may damage surfaces. If an inadequate disinfectant is used, infection may follow. The selection of an appropriate disinfectant is therefore a compromise between efficacy, surface compatibility and user friendliness. It may be that, in future, more emphasis will be placed on cleansing and the selection of less irritant and more environmentally friendly alternatives.

Disinfectants are much more likely to be effective if organic material is removed first. Some disinfectants, e.g. alcohol and glutaraldehyde, are

Table 11.2 Instrument and environmental disinfectants: properties

Disinfectant	Microbicidal activity					Stable	Inactivation by organic matter	Corrosive/ damaging	Irritant/ sensitizing
	Spores	Mycobacteria	Bacteria	Viruses					
				Env	Non-Env				
Glutaraldehyde 2%	Good (slow)	Good (slow)	Good	Good	Good	Moderately (e.g. 14–28 days)	No (fixative)	No	Yes
Peracetic acid 0.2–0.35%	Good	Good	Good	Good	Good	No (1 day)	No	Slight	Slight
Alcohol 60–85%	None	Good	Good	Good	Moderate	Yes	Yes (fixative)	Slight (lens cements)	No (flammable)
Peroxygen compounds*	None	Poor	Good	Good	Moderate	Moderately (e.g. 7 days)	Yes	Slight	No
Chlorine-releasing agents > 1000 ppm av Cl*	Good	Good	Good	Good	Good	No (1 day)	Yes	Yes	Yes
Clear soluble phenolics 0.6–2%	None	Good	Good	Good	Poor	Yes	No	Slight	Yes
Quaternary ammonium compounds*	None	Variable	Moderate	Moderate	Poor	Yes	Yes	No	No

* Activity varies with concentration of product.

fixatives and if intricate or lumened devices are not cleaned first, blockage and instrument malfunction may occur. In addition to inactivation by organic material, some disinfectants are neutralized by soap, hard water, cork and plastics. Disinfectants may also damage surfaces, instrument components and the skin. It is therefore essential that the disinfectant used is compatible with the items and surfaces processed, if irritant substances are used, gloves should be worn and all traces of the disinfectant removed before the item is reused.

Most policies include a disinfectant together with an alternative for each application, i.e. heat-sensitive instruments, spillage and the skin.

Disinfectant testing

Unfortunately, in many countries there are no recognized standard tests for antiseptics and disinfectants, no register of approved products and no centralized funding to ensure the impartiality of test centres. Approval of new disinfectants is fraught with problems. It is hoped that these difficulties will eventually be resolved in Europe, as the EU is currently formulating standard test procedures. However, in the meantime, it would seem reasonable to test all new products alongside existing disinfectants used for the same purpose. Evaluations should be carried out using suspension and carrier tests in the presence/absence of a suitable organic load. A wide range of test organisms should be selected which meet the user's requirements and substantiate manufacturers' efficacy claims. Specific pathogens, or safe surrogates, may be used. At least a 5 $\log_{10}$ reduction (99.999%) is normally required to qualify disinfection.

It is usual to include Gram-positive and Gram-negative bacteria, fungi and viruses. Mycobacteria, e.g. *Mycobacterium tuberculosis* or *M. terrae*, are often included as particularly stringent test organisms, and if destroyed, are indicative of high-level disinfection. If a sterility claim is made, a sporing organism, e.g. *Bacillus subtilis* var *niger*, should be used. As there is little or no legislation which prevents the sale of ineffective disinfectants, purchasers are advised to seek independent reports which substantiate manufacturers' claims. The application and properties of several widely used disinfectants for instruments, the environment and the skin will be described here.

Instruments disinfectants

Only reusable, heat-sensitive instruments and equipment should be processed using disinfectants (Ayliffe *et al.* 1992b, 1993).

Aldehydes

Two per cent glutaraldehyde, e.g. Cidex, Asep, Totacide is the most widely used instrument disinfectant. Other aldehydes, such as succine dialdehyde and formaldehyde (i.e. Gigasept), are occasionally used. Glutaraldehyde has a wide spectrum of antimicrobial activity, but is only slowly effective against mycobacteria and spores. It is non-corrosive and does not damage rubber, lens cements, plastics and other instrument components. Because of its compatibility and efficacy qualities, it is the principal disinfectant for flexible endoscopes which do not tolerate thermal disinfection or sterilization (Babb, 1993a). Unfortunately the aldehydes are toxic, irritant and sensitizing and, as such, have become a principal target for risk assessment and hazard control, e.g. COSHH regulations, in the UK. Suitable gloves, e.g. nitrile and fluid-proof protective clothing should be worn, immersion tanks covered, instruments thoroughly rinsed and toxic vapours suitably contained or extracted. The use of automated washer disinfectors is preferred and further reduces staff exposure (British Society of Gastroenterology Working Party, 1993).

Immersion times vary depending on the nature of microbial contamination anticipated. Most non-sporing bacteria and viruses are killed within 5 min, but some mycobacteria, e.g. *M. tuberculosis*, are more tolerant and take 20 min or more. The *Bacillus subtilis* spores used to validate sterility claims are extremely tolerant to glutaraldehyde and 3–10 h immersion is usually recommended by the disinfectant manufacturers. This is impractical for most users and contact times of 10–20 min are normally used. In the UK, the disinfectant manufacturers, professional societies and the Department of Health have produced guidelines on disinfectant contact times after a careful risk assessment (Medical Devices Agency, 1996). Users are advised to follow these guidelines where practical. Independent testing of disinfectants, with published results, should be carried out before recommendations are made.

Peracetic acid

Peracetic acid, i.e. 0.35% NuCidex and 0.2% Steris (used at 45–50°C), have recently been introduced as less irritant alternatives to glutaraldehyde (Bradley *et al.*, 1995; Babb and Bradley, 1995a). Peracetic acid is highly effective as a microbicide and tests with *B. subtilis* spores confirm sterilant claims following immersion for 10 min. Other non-sporing bacteria, including mycobacteria and viruses are killed in 5 min (Lynam *et al.*, 1995; Holton *et al.* 1994; Griffiths *et al.*, 1998). Unfortunately the disinfectant is less stable and more expensive than glutaraldehyde. It also appears to damage, on prolonged contact, copper alloys and the components of some instruments and processing equipment in spite of the use of a corrosion inhibitor. It is, however, one of the most rapid and efficacious alternatives to glutaraldehyde.

Chlorine dioxide

Another recently introduced instrument disinfectant is chlorine dioxide (Tristel, 1100 ppm av ClO_2). This is also a highly effective disinfectant and its spectrum of activity is similar to peracetic acid. It is also an irritant and damages some instrument components and processing equipment. Its suitability for endoscopes is therefore still under scrutiny.

Alcohol

Alcohol (60–80% ethanol or isopropanol) is another widely used instrument and surface disinfectant. It is a much safer product than the aldehydes and is recommended where no or little provision has been made for personal protection or vapour control. It is also popular as a skin disinfectant. Alcohol destroys most non-sporing bacteria and viruses in under 10 min on clean surfaces. Its principal advantage is that it rapidly evaporates, leaving surfaces dry. Rinsing to remove toxic residues is therefore unnecessary. Consequently it is useful for disinfecting items that are heat sensitive and required rapidly, such as thermometers, trolley tops, meat temperature probes, speculae, scissors and dropped surgical instruments. Alcohol is also useful for wiping over electrical equipment which cannot be immersed. The principal problems associated with alcohol are its flammability and incompatibility with some optical lens cements.

Other agents

Peroxygen compounds, e.g. Virkon, and quartenary ammonium compounds, e.g. Dettol ED and Sactimed Sinald, are occasionally used for instrument disinfection. These are often good cleansing agents and are more user friendly. However, efficacy tests with spores, mycobacteria and some viruses have proved disappointing. These less efficacious agents should be considered when a non-damaging or more user-friendly product is required and where the risk of infection with disinfectant-tolerant organisms is unlikely.

If it is decided to use one of these new glutaraldehyde alternatives, it is recommended that the instrument and processing equipment manufacturers are informed, as use may invalidate guarantees. It is also important that the change is costed, bearing in mind the use life of the disinfectant, ventilation if required and protective clothing (Babb and Bradley, 1995a). It is essential that items are cleaned first, that the manufacturers' stated contact times are achieved and that those responsible for producing disinfectant policy are kept informed of progress, be it favourable or not.

Medical equipment

Medical equipment is often brought into close contact with a susceptible site on the patient or member of staff and infection can occur if the equipment has not been properly decontaminated after previous use. These infection risks have increased in recent years because of more susceptible patients and the increasing use of heat-labile equipment which is often difficult to clean and disinfect, e.g. flexible fibreoptic endoscopes (Ayliffe, 1988). Nevertheless, infection from equipment is infrequent due to improved methods of decontamination and well-trained staff, especially sterile service departments.

The selection of the most appropriate decontamination method depends on many factors, but especially on the infection risk to the patient (see Chapter 9).

Endoscopes

Endoscopy has increased in recent years for both diagnostic and operative procedures. Many operations, e.g. cholecystectomy, are now carried out using minimal access surgery. Operative endoscopes, e.g. laparoscopes and arthroscopes, are in the high-infection risk category and should be sterilized. They are mainly rigid and can usually be autoclaved. If heat labile they can be sterilized by ethylene oxide or immersion in 2% glutaraldehyde, although in practice it is usually not possible for endoscopes and accessories as these processes do not allow sufficient time for treatment between patients during an operating session. Disinfection with 2% glutaraldehyde, i.e. exposure for 10–20 min, is mainly used and although some spores are not killed by this process there is little evidence of infection caused by spore-bearing organisms (Ayliffe *et al.*, 1992a). Few spores or other organisms, including viruses, remain on an endoscope after thorough cleaning (Hanson *et al.*, 1990; Babb and Bradley, 1995b).

Infections occurring after endoscopic surgery are mainly endogenous or from the operator and not from equipment. Newer agents, e.g. peracetic acid, chlorine dioxide and superoxidized water, are sporicidal in less than 10 min and, if otherwise acceptable, might be alternative sterilizing agents in the future (Babb and Bradley, 1995a). Flexible endoscopes, e.g. gastroscopes, colonoscopes and bronchoscopes, are included in the intermediate infection risk category and require disinfection after cleaning (see Chapter 9). They are heat labile and gastrointestinal endoscopes have long narrow channels (suction, biopsy, water, air, CO_2) which are difficult to clean (Babb, 1993a).

Infections from these endoscopes have mainly been due to opportunist Gram-negative bacilli, e.g. *Ps. aeruginosa*, *Klebsiella* spp., *Serratia marcescens* and *Acinetobacter* spp. These organisms grow overnight in the moist conditions within the channels of the endoscope and in the water-bottle and processing equipment. They may cause respiratory infections or more commonly cholangitis and septicaemia following ERCP. Occasional outbreaks of salmonella have been reported following gastroscopy (Spach *et al.*, 1993; Ayliffe, 1996). Transmission of tuberculosis from bronchoscopes has rarely been reported (e.g. Leers, 1980), only one well-documented case of hepatitis B (Birnie *et al.*, 1983) and no cases of HIV. Most of these cases have been due to inadequate cleaning or the use of inappropriate disinfectants, e.g. hexachlorophane or quaternary ammonium compounds, and few have been described in recent years since the introduction of national guidelines (British Society of Gastroenterology, 1998; Medical Devices Agency, 1996). Mycobacteria, e.g. *Myco. chelonae* have been responsible for occasional infections or pseudoepidemics following bronchoscopy. These organisms have been isolated from the rinse water, tanks and pipework of washer disinfectors and grow in biofilms (Babb and Bradley, 1995b). Some of these environmentally associated mycobacteria are resistant to glutaraldehyde (Griffiths *et al.*, 1997). Disinfecting washer disinfectors and water-treatment facilities with a chlorine-releasing agent or peracetic acid, rinsing the bronchoscope channel with 70% alcohol and allowing to dry will further reduce the chances of survival of Gram-negative bacilli and atypical mycobacteria.

Two per cent glutaraldehyde remains the disinfectant of choice for endosope disinfection (Ayliffe, 1993), but it is irritant and toxic. Exhaust ventilation must be provided to keep levels of glutaraldehyde in the air at an acceptable level (British Society of Gastroenterology Working Party, 1993). The newer agents described above rapidly kill non-sporing bacteria

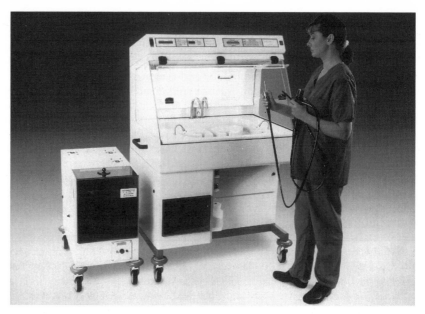

Figure 11.2   A modern flexible endoscope washer disinfector with a filtration system for removing bacteria from the rinse water

and inactivate viruses and are microbiologically suitable for endoscope disinfection but all have potential problems (Babb and Bradley, 1995b). Further in-use studies are necessary before replacing glutaraldehyde, which has been in use for many years.

Automated chemical washer/disinfectors for endoscopes

Several automated machines are now available which can be programmed to clean, disinfect and rinse the internal channels and external surfaces of flexible fibreoptic endoscopes and their accessories (Figure 11.2). Studies have shown that this equipment can offer a more reliable decontamination process than can be achieved manually. They also contribute towards reducing skin contact with irritant disinfectants like glutaraldehyde, the disinfectant most widely used for endoscopes (Bradley and Babb, 1995).

When purchasing equipment, it is more important to establish that it is effective, non-damaging, safe and is sufficiently versatile to accommodate the various types of endoscopes used. It should also enable the user to select a suitable disinfectant contact time which will meet the requirements of national or local policies (Medical Devices Agency, 1966). All-channel irrigation is important, so too is a final rinse. The rinse water must be of good microbiological quality and preferably sterile or passed through a bacteria-retaining filter (0.2–0.45 μm). This is particularly important for invasive endoscopes and bronchoscopes. As washer disinfectors may acquire micro-organisms from patients via endoscopes or the environment, it is important that they are put through a self-disinfect cycle which will ensure all immersion and storage tanks, water treatment and associated pipe work are disinfected. This should be done at the start of each session.

A number of other considerations should be taken into account when selecting a washer disinfector. For example, is a fixed or mobile unit required; is there a cycle counter and fault indicator; is more than one endoscope to be processed, and if so is synchronous or asynchronous processing required; is there a printout of cycle parameters?

Disinfectants rapidly become diluted in automated systems due to carry-over of water or detergent. It is therefore important to establish when to change the disinfectant. If 2% glutaraldehyde is used it is recommended that the concentration does not fall below 1.5%. Transfer of disinfectant to the rinse water and then to the endoscope also occurs, thus increasing the risk of irritancy to the patient or instrument user. The rinse water should therefore be changed frequently, preferably after each cycle. Pumping air through the channels will express residual water, but effective drying will only occur with hot air or alcohol. Storing a dry instrument will decrease the likelihood of microbial proliferation during storage.

Several new machines now have an integral aldehyde vapour-handling system which either extract to the outside or recirculate vapour through a dedicated glutaraldehyde absorbent charcoal filter. These are much preferred, as they reduce staff exposure to aldehyde fumes.

Periodic testing may be necessary to ensure that the washer disinfector is functioning correctly and that the machine and rinse water do not become a source of recontamination which may put the patient at risk or jeopardize the diagnostic and operative function of the instrument.

Respiratory equipment

Lower respiratory infection is a common complication of mechanical ventilation, but the organisms are mainly endogenous in origin (see Chapter 5). However, infection can occur from contaminated medical devices (Das and Fraise, 1997). The main organisms transferred from equipment are opportunist Gram-negative bacilli, e.g. *Pseudomonas aeruginosa*, *Klebsiella* spp., *Serratia marcescens* and *Acinetobacter* spp. These organisms will grow overnight in residual moisture and soil in inadequately decontaminated equipment or in equipment containing water. Although contamination of respiratory equipment is often reported, clinical infection due to inadequately decontaminated respiratory medical devices is rare, in recent years.

Pseudomonas infection acquired from a contaminated ventilator has been reported (Phillips and Spencer, 1966) and acinetobacter infection from contaminated ventilator tubing (Cefai *et al.*, 1990). Aerosols containing pseudomonas have caused pneumonia (Reinarz *et al.*, 1965). *Mycobacterium tuberculosis* has been isolated from anaesthetic face masks (Livingstone *et al.*, 1941), but there is surprisingly little evidence of spread of infection.

Respiratory equipment is an intermediate infection risk and disinfection after cleaning should be adequate, but autoclaving is preferred if the items are not damaged by the process. Thermal disinfection of the ventilator circuit in a washer disinfector is the usual method used but, if pasteurization is not possible, disinfection with a chlorine-releasing agent (125–500 ppm of available chlorine) is a less satisfactory alternative. Thorough cleaning is particularly important and so is rinsing after chemical disinfection. The outside of machines can be disinfected by wiping with 70% alcohol.

In patients on long-term ventilation, changing the circuit every 48–72 h is commonly recommended. Ventilators are difficult to clean and disinfect and filters are usually used to protect the machine from contamination. This removes the need for routine disinfection, but disinfection can be carried out with formaldehyde if required (Ayliffe *et al.*, 1992b). Some ventilators have autoclavable internal circuits.

Heat moisturisers reduce the amount of condensate and this reduces the frequency of changing the circuit, especially in neonates (Cadwallader *et al.*, 1990). Humidifiers should be changed every 48 h, cleaned and dried and preferably disinfected by heat. Some can be disinfected by raising the temperature of the water in the humidifier to over 70°C.

Anaesthetic machines and circuits present less of a contamination problem since they are only used on a single patient for a relatively short time (du Moulin and Saubeman, 1977), but if untreated, opportunist Gram-negative bacilli will grow overnight. On the other hand, there is a risk of cross-infection between patients on an operating list, but this appears to be uncommon provided that each patient has a clean and disinfected face mask and connection or endotracheal tube. A recent report has suggested the possible spread of hepatitis C between patients on an operating list mediated by anaesthetic equipment (Ragg, 1994). The circumstantial evidence is strong, but transfer of infection by another route such as a contaminated syringe cannot be ruled out. Although it is preferable from the micro-biological aspect to provide each patient with a clean circuit for an operation, this is expensive and not cost effective. A sessional exchange system, e.g. a clean circuit after every 9 or 10 operations, would appear to be microbiologically acceptable (Deverill and Dutt, 1980). It has been suggested that a filter, changed after every patient, would be cheaper than reprocessing a circuit, but there is little evidence that infection would be reduced (Das and Fraise, 1997). Disposable circuits are often preferred since they are less heavy than reusables, but they are expensive. There are some possible indications for their use, e.g. on a patient with pulmonary tuberculosis.

There are other items of respiratory equipment which are difficult to clean and disinfect, e.g. spirometers. Most have been designed without considering the need for decontamination. Each item must be considered separately, but at least a disposable mouthpiece should be used. It is advisable to use an inexpensive filter for each series of patient tests, particularly if air is expired and inspired through respiratory function equipment and provided that this does not affect the diagnostic result.

The environment

The routine disinfection of ward floors and other surfaces remote from the patient is wasteful, unnecessary and often damaging (see Chapter 8). Provided that floors and horizontal surfaces are cleaned without raising dust and adherent micro-organisms, they are unlikely to become a source of infection as they rarely come into contact with a susceptible site. However, disinfectants are used to protect staff while removing potentially hazardous material such as spilt blood, body fluids, cultures and other infectious materials from

Table 11.3 Some uses of chlorine-releasing agents and solution strengths

Organic load	Task	Available chlorine	
		(%)	(ppm)
High	Blood spills	1.0	10,000
	Laboratory discard	0.25	2.500
Medium	Precleaned surfaces	0.1	1,000
Low	Precleaned medical equipment, e.g. tonometers, respiratory and catering equipment	0.020–0.05	200–500
	Infant feed bottles	0.0125	125
Extremely low	Hydrotherapy pools		4–6
	Drinking water		0.5–1

environmental surfaces. If such material is left on the surface it may prove slippery, offensive and a potential source of transmission.

Disinfectants are also used for decontaminating cleaning equipment and environmental surfaces (Babb, 1996) which are in contact with the skin of infected patients or those colonized with multi-resistant or highly communicable micro-organisms such as methicillin-resistant *Staph. aureus* (MRSA), vancomycin-resistant enterococci (VRE) or *Clostridium difficile*.

Chlorine-releasing agents

The most widely used agents for inanimate surfaces are the chlorine-releasing agents, e.g. sodium hypochlorite (bleach NaOCl) or sodium dichloro-isocyanurate (NaDCC) (Ayliffe *et al.*, 1993). These are used for body fluid spills, laboratory discard, bench tops, kitchen work surfaces, infant feeding bottles, catering equipment, tonometers, dialysers and occasionally for water treatment and respiratory equipment. NaDCC is available as tablets, granules or powders and some contain a compatible detergent. These agents are preferred to sodium hypochlorite because they are easier to prepare and use, are slightly more efficacious and are less damaging to surfaces.

Chlorine-releasing agents are comparatively inexpensive and, if used at a sufficiently high concentration, are rapidly effective against a wide range of micro-organisms including the bloodborne viruses, mycobacteria and bacterial spores. Chlorine-releasing agents are inactivated by organic material and high concentrations, e.g. 5000–10 000 ppm av Cl are recommended for application to body fluid spills or grossly contaminated surfaces (Table 11.3). Chlorine-releasing agents are also corrosive to metals, and damage rubber and some other materials. This damage may be reduced if surfaces are cleaned first and a lower concentration used, i.e. 200–1000 ppm av Cl.

Chlorine-releasing agents should not be diluted in hot water or be mixed with acids, e.g. cleaning solutions and urine, as a rapid release of chlorine may occur which could irritate the eyes and respiratory mucosa of the user. Small spills of blood, i.e. less than 30 ml, and other body fluids are best removed by applying granules or powder directly to the spill. This can then be removed using one or more paper towels. This would, however, be impractical for larger spills which should first be removed and a lower concentration used, i.e. 1000 ppm av Cl. Tablets, granules and powders are all very stable but once prepared at 'in use' concentrations in solution should be used within 24 h. Chlorine-releasing agents are also useful for disinfecting mops and other reusable cleaning equipment if heat treatment is impractical.

Clear soluble phenolics

These are also useful for removing body fluid spills and disinfecting environmental surfaces. Many contain a compatible detergent and cleaning may therefore accompany disinfection. Phenolics are now used less frequently as their virucidal activity is poor. They are not therefore advised for blood spills, particularly if HIV or HBV is suspected. They are, however, highly effective in destroying mycobacteria and other non-sporing bacteria, especially if present in faeces and sputum. Phenolics are comparatively inexpensive but are irritant, taint food and damage some plastics. They are, therefore, unsuitable for the skin, mattresses covers and kitchen surfaces. Concentrations of 0.6–2% are usually advised, depending on the formulation and amount of organic matter present.

Other agents

Other disinfectants suitable for environmental surfaces are the quartenary ammonium compounds, peroxygen compounds and iodophores. These are used for cleaning and disinfecting, especially in kitchens and other areas where the chlorine-releasing agents and phenolics cannot be used because they taint food or damage equipment. Their spectrum of activity, particularly against mycobacteria, spores and non-enveloped viruses, are poor and they are not advised for high- or intermediate-risk items. Most are, however, excellent cleaning agents and are more user friendly than many of the more efficacious disinfectants.

Fogging is an ineffective means of disinfecting the air and surfaces, and may lead to the inhalation of toxic substances. Ventilating the room and applying a suitable disinfectant to the surfaces with friction is likely to be safer and more effective in clinical areas.

Skin and mucous membranes

The purpose of skin disinfection is: to protect open wounds and other vulnerable sites from micro-organisms transferred on the hands of staff, to protect the patient's tissues against his/her endogenous flora during surgery or an invasive technique, and occasionally to treat carriers and dispersers of multi-resistant strains, e.g. MRSA.

The normal skin flora consists mainly of Gram-positive, coagulase-negative, cocci, e.g. *Staph. epidermidis*, other staphylococci, and aerobic and anaerobic diphtheroids. These are known as residents and rarely cause infection, apart from their introduction during invasive procedures, e.g. surgery or insertion of intravenous lines. The resident skin flora grows naturally on the skin and is difficult to remove by normal skin-cleansing techniques (Lowbury, 1992).

Micro-organisms acquired or deposited on the skin from other patients, staff or the inanimate environment are known as transients. These are unlikely to grow on the skin and are readily removed or destroyed by thorough cleaning or disinfection. The transient flora includes most of the micro-organisms responsible for cross-infection, e.g. *Staph. aureus*, *Escherichia coli*, *Pseudomonas aeruginosa*, *Salmonella* spp. and rotaviruses.

Hands

The hands are considered to be one of the principal routes of spread of infection. Effective handwashing or disinfection is probably the most important infection control measure. It is not unusual to find one-third of the nursing staff carrying transient organisms on their hands at any one time and this increases during outbreaks, following contact with grossly contaminated surfaces or during lapses in compliance with handwashing and disinfection procedures (Ayliffe *et al.*, 1988). Numbers of transients recovered from the hands can be as high as 10^{10}, although 10^3–10^4 is more common.

The transient and resident skin flora can be removed or destroyed by the application of soap and water, antiseptic soaps and detergents or alcoholic handrubs. Transients are superficial and more easily removed or destroyed than residents which colonize the hair follicles and deeper layers and crevices of the skin. Reasons why, how and when health care staff should wash or disinfect their hands are summarized in Tables 11.4 and 11.5. Washing with bar or liquid soap and water removes dirt, rendering the hands socially clean. Provided that it is done thoroughly, it also removes in the order of 99% of transient flora. This will normally suffice for wards, kitchens and most clinical areas. Liquid soaps usually contain a bacteriostatic agent which prevents microbial proliferation during storage and use.

Many antiseptic formulations are more effective in removing or destroying transient micro-organisms than non-medicated soap. They are preferred where the risks of hand transmission are greater, e.g. in neonatal, isolation and intensive care units, during outbreaks of infection or for procedures where contact with body fluids is likely. Some, such as chlorhexidine and triclosan, have a residual effect which sustains antimicrobial activity so that micro-organisms subsequently deposited on the skin are less likely to survive. If a thorough technique is used, the more effective antiseptic soaps and detergents, e.g. those containing chlorhexidine or povidone-iodine, will enhance killing of transient bacteria by approximately 1 $\log_{10}$, i.e. 99–99.9% (Ayliffe *et al.*, 1988).

The application of alcohol in solution, or as a gel or foam, does not remove micro-organisms but rapidly destroys them on the skin surfaces. Studies have shown that some alcohols (i.e. 60–80% isopropanol or ethanol) are even more effective than aqueous antiseptic soaps and detergents but are only suitable for clean hands. Alcohol hand-rubs are particularly valuable

Table 11.4   Why, how and when to handwash

	Social handwash	Hygienic hand disinfection	Surgical scrub
Why	Use a bar or liquid soap to render the hands socially clean and remove transient micro-organisms	Use antiseptics to remove or destroy all/most transient micro-organisms. A residual effect is preferable	Use antiseptics to remove/destroy transient micro-organisms and substantially reduce detachable resident micro-organisms. A prolonged effect is required
How	A thorough wash with a cosmetically acceptable bar or liquid soap	A thorough defined wash for 15–30 s with an antiseptic soap or detergent, e.g. chlorhexidine, povidone-iodine or triclosan. Alternatively, apply an alcohol hand-rub to disinfect clean hands	Scrape/brush nails and apply antiseptic soap or detergent, e.g. chlorhexidine or povidone-iodine, to hands and forearms using a defined technique for a minimum of 2 min. Dry hands on a sterile towel. Alternatively, clean hands with soap and water and apply two or more applications of an alcohol hand-rub
When	All routine tasks within general wards and catering establishments	During outbreaks of infection, in high-risk areas, when contact with infectious material is likely or at the discretion of the Infection Control Committee	Prior to surgery or invasive procedures, at the discretion of the Infection Control Committee

Table 11.5   Examples of when to wash or disinfect hands

Before
- Aseptic procedures, e.g. catheterization, dressing change
- Surgical procedures and injections
- Entering isolation rooms
- Preparing food

After
- Leaving source isolation
- Contact with secretions and excretions
- Using the lavatory, handling bedpans and urine bottles
- Cleaning duties and bed making

in areas devoid of running water or where return to a wash basin is impractical, e.g. in the community or during a ward round. An emollient incorporated with the rub, e.g. glycerol, is necessary to prevent the hands from drying and chapping.

A high proportion of surgical gloves are punctured or damaged by bone splinters, needles or sharp instruments during surgery. In one study the clean wound postoperative infection rate increased threefold when the gloves became damaged. However, this has not been confirmed in subsequent studies. It is therefore logical to use antiseptic formulations which are highly effective in removing or destroying bacteria which would otherwise pass through holes in the gloves increasing infection risk. Effective antiseptic detergent scrubs, e.g. those containing chlorhexidine, povidone-iodine, or alcoholic hand-rubs, are therefore recommended prior to surgery. Products with a prolonged effect are preferred to give lasting protection under the gloves. Sterile nail brushes or sticks may be used to clean nails prior to the first operation of the day, but are rarely required at other times. Frequent use of nail brushes damages the skin and may increase microbial proliferation. Hands should be dried on a sterile towel before donning gloves.

The activity of antiseptics varies with the formulation and nature of contamination. The efficacy of formulations for hygienic hand disinfection are usually assessed by measuring a reduction in transient flora, e.g. *E. coli* artificially applied to the hands or fingertips. The most efficacious agents are those containing 60–80% isopropanol or ethanol, 4% chlorhexidine gluconate and 7.5% povidone-iodine. Surgical scrubs are usually assessed using a glove juice technique by measuring their immediate and prolonged effect (3 h) on the resident skin flora (Babb *el al.*, 1991). Although the rank order of effectiveness is similar to products for hygienic hand disinfection, the reductions in resident flora are less pronounced and no reduction occurs with unmedicated bar soap.

Studies using electronic counting equipment have shown that handwashing frequency is much lower than that claimed. It is essential that detergents and hand-rubs are cosmetically acceptable or they will not be used. The application techniques for soaps, detergents and alcoholic hand-rubs are also poor. A thorough wash, including the fingertips, with an acceptable formulation is more important than using a more effective but damaging formulation. Some examples of when to wash or disinfect the hands are shown in Table 11.6.

Operation site

A rapid reduction in skin flora (transients and residents) is required for the operation site. The most suitable agents are 60–80% isopropanol or ethanol (Lowbury, 1992; Ayliffe *et al.*, 1993). Provided that the skin is clean, they work rapidly and evaporate leaving the surface dry. The addition of other agents such as dyes, 0.5% chlorhexidine, 1% iodine or 10% povidone-iodine (now preferred to iodine as it causes fewer skin reactions) may help to identify treated areas and may prolong the antimicrobial effect, but they do not appear to enhance significantly the immediate effect. Antiseptics should be applied to the skin with friction. This is more effectively done in the theatre after shaving or clipping and immediately prior to surgery.

There is little evidence to support the use of antiseptics for disinfection of mucous membranes. Alcoholic formulations are usually too painful to apply but have been used in the mouth prior to dental surgery. Antiseptics are soon diluted or inactivated by saliva, mucus and other body fluids and consequently have only a marginal effect. Chlorhexidine 0.2% mouthwashes are available for oral hygiene and these have been used for the treatment and prevention of gingivitis.

The urethra normally has few commensal bacteria but is liable to become contaminated on passage of a catheter or instruments. A solution of 0.02% chlorhexidine instilled into the urethra, or applied with lignocaine, will disinfect the meatus prior to cystocopy or catheterization. Cleaning with dilute Savlon or Savlodil (chlorhexidine 0.015% and cetrimide 0.15%) or a vaginal douche with 0.5% povidone-iodine followed by the use of 10% povidone-iodine gel, can be used for the vaginal mucosa. An obstetric cream containing 1% chlorhexidine gluconate may be used as an antiseptic lubricant during vaginal examinations.

Reference and further reading

Ayliffe, G.A.J. (1988) Equipment related infection risks. *J. Hosp. Infect.*, **11** (suppl. A), 279–284.

Ayliffe, G.A.J. (1993) Principles of cleaning and disinfection: which disinfectant? *Infection in Endoscopy, Gastrointest. Clin. N. Am.*, **3**, 411–429.

Ayliffe, G.A.J. (1996) Nosocomial infections associated with endoscopy. In *Hospital Epidemiology and Infection Control* (C.G. Mayhall, ed.), Baltimore, Williams and Wilkins.

Ayliffe, G.A.J., Babb, J.R., Davies, J.G. and Lilly, H.A. (1988) Hand disinfection: a comparison of various agents in laboratory and ward studies. *J. Hosp. Infect.*, **11**, 226–243.

Ayliffe, G.A.J., Babb, J.R. and Bradley, C.R. (1992a) Sterilization of arthroscopes and laparoscopes. *J. Hosp. Infect.*, **22**, 265–269.

Ayliffe, G.A.J., Lowbury, E.J.L., Geddes, A.M. and Williams, J.D. (1992b) *Control of Hospital Infection: A Practical Handbook*, 3rd edn, London, Chapman and Hall.

Ayliffe, G.A.J., Coates, D. and Hoffman, P.N. (1993) *Chemical Disinfection in Hospitals*, London, Public Health Laboratory Service.

Babb, J.R. (1993a) Disinfection and sterilization of endoscopes. *Curr. Opin. Infect. Dis.*, **6**, 532–537.

Babb, J.R. (1993b) Methods of cleaning and disinfection. *Central Sterilization, Central Service*, official publication of the European Society of Hospital Sterile Supply, 227–237.

Babb, J.R. (1996) Application of disinfectants in hospitals and other health care establishments. *Infect. Control J. South. Afr.*, **1**, 4–12.

Babb, J.R. and Bradley, C.R. (1995a) A review of glutaraldehyde alternatives. *Br. J. Theatre Nurs.*, **5**, 20–24.

Babb, J.R. and Bradley, C.R. (1995b) Endoscopy decontamination: where do we go from here? *J. Hosp. Infect.*, **30** (suppl.), 543–551.

Babb, J.R. and Lynam, P. (1993) Process options for biohazards: whether or not to autoclave. *J. Sterile Serv. Manage.*, **4**, 5–9.

Babb, J.R., Bradley, C.R. and Ayliffe, G.A.J. (1982) A formaldehyde disinfection unit. *J. Hosp. Infect.*, **3**, 193–197.

Babb, J.R., Davies, J.G. and Ayliffe, G.A.J. (1991) A test procedure for evaluating surgical hand disinfection. *J. Hosp. Infect.*, **18** (suppl. B), 41–49.

Barrie, D. (1994) Infection control in practice: how hospital linen and laundry services are provided. *J. Hosp. Infect.*, **27**, 219–235.

Birnie, G.G., Quigley, E.M., Clements, G.B. *et al.* (1983) Endoscopic transmission of hepatitis B virus. *Gut*, **24**, 171–174.

Bradley, C.R. and Babb, J.R. (1995) Endoscope decontamination automated vs manual. *J. Hosp. Infect.*, **30** (suppl.), 537–542.

Bradley, C.R. and Babb, J.R. and Ayliffe, G.A.J. (1995) Evaluation of the steris system I Peracetic acid endoscope processor. *J. Hosp. Infect.*, **29**, 143–151.

British Society of Gastroenterology (1998) Cleaning and disinfection of equipment for gastrointestinal flexible endoscopy. Working Party Report. *Gut*, **42**, 583–593.

British Society of Gastroenterology Working Party (1993) Aldehyde disinfectants and health in endoscopy units. Special Report. *Gut*, **34**, 1641–1645.

British Standards Institution (1993) British Standard 2745, Parts 1–3: Washer Disinfections for Medical Purposes. London, British Standards Institution.

Cadwallader, H.L., Bradley, C.R. and Ayliffe, G.A.J. (1990) Bacterial contamination and frequency of changing ventilator circuitry. *J. Hosp. Infect.*, **15**, 65–72.

Cefai, C., Richards, J., Gould, F.K. and McPeake, P. (1990) An outbreak of acinetobacter respiratory tract infection resulting from incomplete disinfection of ventilating equipment. *J. Hosp. Infect.*, **15**, 177–182.

Coates, D. and Hutchinson, D.N. (1994) How to produce a hospital disinfection policy. *J. Hosp. Infect.* **26**, 57–68.

Das, I. and Fraise, A.P. (1997) How useful are microbial filters in respiratory apparatus? *J. Hosp. Infect.*, **37**, 263–272.

Deverill, C.E.A. and Dutt, K.K. (1980) Methods of decontamination of anaesthetic equipment. *J. Hosp. Infect.*, **1**, 165–170.

du Moulin, G.C. and Saubermann, A.J. (1977) The anaesthesia machine and circle system are not likely to be sources of bacterial contamination. *Anaesthesiology*, **47**, 353–358.

Griffiths, P.A., Babb, J.R., Bradley, C.R. and Fraise, A.P. (1997) Glutaraldehyde resistant *Mycobacterium chelonae* from endoscope washer disinfectors. *J. Appl. Microbiol.*, **82**, 519–526.

Griffiths, P.A., Babb, J.R. and Fraise, A.P. (1998) Mycobactericidal activity of selected disinfectants using a quantitative suspension test. *J. Hosp. Infect.* (in press).

Hanson, P.J., Gor, D., Jeffries, D.J. and Collins J.V. (1990) Elimination of 'high titre' HIV from fibre optic endoscopes. *Gut*, **31**, 657–660.

Holton, J., Nye, P. and McDonald, V. (1994) Efficacy of selected disinfectants against mycobacteria and cryptospaudia. *J. Hosp. Infect.* **27**, 105–115.

Leers, W. (1980) Disinfecting endoscopes: how not to transmit *Mycobacterium tuberculosis* by bronchoscopy. *Can. Med. Assoc. J.*, **123**, 275–283.

Livingstone, H., Heidrick, F., Holicky, I. and Dack, G.M. (1941) Cross-infection from anaesthetic face masks. *Surgery*, **9**, 433–435.

Lowbury, E.J.L. (1992) Special problems in antisepsis. In *Principles and Practice of Disinfection, Preservation and Sterilization*, 2nd edn (A.D. Russell, W.B. Hugo and G.A.J. Ayliffe, eds), Oxford, Blackwell.

Lynam, P.A., Babb, J.R. and Fraise, A.P. (1995) Comparison of mycobactericidal activity of 2% alkaline glutaraldehyde and Nu-cidex (0.35% peracetic acid). *J. Hosp. Infect.*, **30**, 237–239.

Medical Devices Agency (1993/96) *Sterilization, Disinfection and Cleaning of Medical Equipment: Guidance on Decontamination. Part 1: Principles*; *Part 2: Protocols*; and *Part 3: Procedures* (in preparation), London, HMSO.

Medical Devices Agency (1996) *Decontamination of Endoscopes*, Device Bulletin 9607, London, Department of Health.

NHS Estates (1995) *Washer Disinfectors*, Health Technical Memorandum 2030, London, HMSO.

Phillips, I. and Spencer, G. (1966) *Pseudomonas aeruginosa* cross-infection due to contaminated respiratory apparatus. *Lancet*, **2**, 1325–1327.

Ragg, M. (1994) Transmission of hepatitis C via anaesthetic tubings. *Lancet*, **343**, 1419.

Reinarz, J.A., Pierce, A.K., Mays, B.B. and Sandford, J.P. (1965) The 'potential' role of inhalation therapy equipment in nosocomial pulmonary infection. *J. Clin. Invest.*, **44**, 831–839.

Rutala, W.A. (1990) APIC guidelines for selection of use of disinfectants. *Am. Med. J. Infect. Cont.*, **18**, 99–117.

Spach, D.H., Silverstein, F.E. and Stamm, W.E. (1993) Transmission of infection by gastrointestinal endoscopy and bronchoscopy. *Ann. Int. Med.*, **18**, 117–128.

12

Sterilization

Sterilization is usually described as the complete destruction or removal of micro-organisms. In practice, defining the required standard is more difficult (Kelsey, 1972), as the size of the load, its tolerance to the process and the speed at which effective penetration of the sterilant occurs must also be considered. If the item is not thoroughly cleaned, or the surfaces are inaccessible, sterilization may not be achieved. Killing 10^6 bacterial spores of a defined resistance to the process is commonly accepted as the standard, i.e. a probability of more than one in a million chance that a resistant spore will survive the process. Although on occasions large numbers of micro-organisms are present on used instruments, many of these will be removed during cleaning and of those that remain, most will be far more susceptible to the sterilant than the spores originally used to validate the process. Autoclaving will usually meet the required standard with a very large margin of safety, but many items are heat sensitive and cannot be processed in this way.

Items that normally require sterilization are those which are invasive, and enter vascular systems or sterile body cavities (Ayliffe *et al.*, 1984). This includes surgical instruments, implants, catheters, needles, syringes, infusions, injections, surgical swabs, dressings and sutures. Items sterilized and not immediately used are usually packaged or contained to protect them from recontamination during storage. Problems are most likely to occur when sterilizing heat-sensitive items. These are usually processed in hospitals using liquid or gaseous sterilants. Thorough cleaning, and ensuring that the sterilant comes into contact with all contaminated surfaces, is essential as is the removal of toxic residues by aeration or rinsing in sterile water. Sometimes, no practical or local means of sterilization is available for heat-sensitive items, e.g. flexible endoscopes, in which case high-level disinfection becomes the objective.

The various options for sterilizing heat-tolerant and heat-sensitive items are shown in Table 12.1.

Steam sterilization: autoclave

Autoclaving is the most effective and least problematic method of sterilization. Steam under pressure attains temperatures above 100°C and this is usually sufficient to destroy micro-organisms, including bacterial spores.

Table 12.1   Sterilization: process options for clean reusable items

Process	Cycle parameters
Heat-tolerant items	
Steam sterilization	
Autoclaves:	
porous load	134–138°C for 3 min
unwrapped instruments	121–124°C for 15 min
transportable (bench top)	or 134–138°C for 3 min
bottled fluids	115°C for 30 min
	or 121°C for 15 min
Hot air oven	180°C for 30 min
	170°C for 1 h
	160°C for 2 h
Heat-sensitive items	
Ethylene oxide	37–55°C up to 6 h
Low-temperature steam and formaldehyde	73–80°C up to 3 h
Gas plasma, e.g. from hydrogen peroxide	45°C for 50–72 min
Sporicidal disinfectants:	
2% glutaraldehyde	Immersion for: 3–10 h
0.2–0.35% peracetic acid	10 min
1000–10 000 ppm av. chlorine or chlorine dioxide	10 min

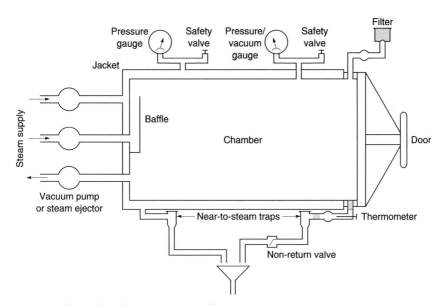

Figure 12.1   Steam pressure sterilizer (autoclave) showing basic features

An autoclave (Figure 12.1) is a pressure vessel supplied with, or generating, steam which is held at a constant pressure for a set time. The process requires direct contact between pure, dry, saturated steam (i.e. at phase boundary conditions) and the item to be sterilized. This must reach the required temperature, for the required time, in the absence of air. The recommended time and temperatures used are those produced by a working

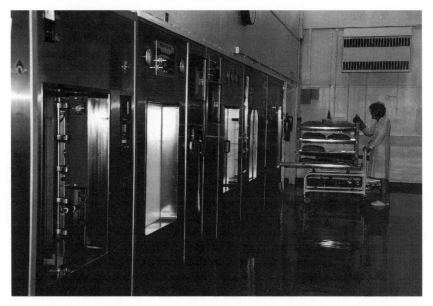

Figure 12.2   Porous load and a low-temperature steam and formaldehyde sterilizer in a hospital
sterilization unit

group of the Medical Research Council in 1959. The cycles most frequently
used in the UK are 121–124°C for 15 min or 134–138°C for 3 min (Medical
Devices Agency, 1993/96).

Autoclaves vary in sophistication, from simple transportable or bench
top sterilizers and pressure cookers, where air is displaced by steam, to
highly sophisticated porous load autoclaves (Figure 12.2) which incorporate
a vacuum-assisted air-removal stage before steam admission. These are
suitable for narrow-lumened devices, packaged instruments and porous loads
such as dressings, swabs and theatre clothing. These porous load autoclaves
are far more expensive than transportable or downward-displacement
autoclaves and are usually installed in sterile services departments where
the throughput justifies it and where they can be suitably maintained and
cycles monitored.

Some autoclaves are suitable for sterilizing bottled fluids. These have
facilities for processing at lower temperatures and for rapid cooling without
losing the bottle contents. Large-chambered downward-displacement
autoclaves without vacuum pumps are also available for unwrapped
instruments and holloware. These are most suited to processing items
immediately prior to reuse, e.g. in operating theatres. Details of the various
types of sterilizers, together with maintenance and process validation and
verification, are given in *British Standard 3970* (1990), NHS Estates *Health
Technical Memorandum 2010* (1994–5); and *MDA Device Bulletin 9605*
(1997); NHS Estates, 1994/95; Medical Devices Agency, 1993–96.

Care should be taken when loading the chamber to ensure that optimum
sterilizing conditions are met. Each sterilizer should be validated for the
particular load for which it is designed. Autoclaves are either supplied with

piped steam or steam is generated by heating water within the sterilizer. Pressure vessels are potentially dangerous and safety locks must be fitted to prevent access to the load while the vessel is still under pressure. Sterilizers for bottled fluids have safety interlocks which prevent access if the contents are at a temperature greater than 80°C, because above this temperature bottles may explode.

A typical cycle of a transportable steam sterilizer for those who do not have access to a sterile services department, e.g. GPs, dentists, chiropodists, etc. (British Medical Association, 1989, British Dental Association, 1996) is as follows. Water is added to the steam generator and this is heated to produce steam; this displaces air which is vented from the chamber until the correct sterilizing temperature is reached. This will depend on the pressure attained. The greater the pressure the higher the temperature. Steam is then held in the chamber for the minimum hold time before it is either exhausted or allowed to condense. The cycle is complete once the pressure has fallen to atmospheric. The lid may then safely be opened. It is preferred that the steam sterilizer has an indicator which informs the user when faults occur and the cycle is complete. Also the sterilizing parameters, i.e. time, chamber temperature and pressure, should be displayed to confirm that the cycle stages have been met.

Performance tests should periodically be undertaken with thermocouples in accordance with national policy. In the UK, BS 3970 and HTM 2010 are available for guidance. Biological indicators (spore tests) are no longer recommended for verification of sterilization but have been used for confirmation if cycle parameters are difficult to measure or have not been met, particularly when no alternative means of sterilization is available. Chemical indicators are useful in identifying processed items. These may be in the form of paper strips, tapes or incorporated into packaging materials. Chemical indicator strips are particularly useful if placed in the processing trays of unwrapped instrument or transportable sterilizers, as they are the only means of indicating that the instruments have been processed after removal from the chamber.

Porous load sterilizers are fitted with air detectors to monitor air removal. In addition to this, a Bowie–Dick test or alternative is required at the beginning of each working day. In this test a cross of autoclave tape on a sheet of paper is placed in the centre of a standard pack of porous material (towels in the original test) and processed. Uniform intensity of the dark stripes the entire length of both sections of the tape indicates adequate air removal. Towel packs vary in thickness, moisture content and absorbency with age and laundering. More reproducible testpieces, e.g. Lantor Cube (3M) and TST single use Bowie–Dick Type Test Pack (Browne), which simulate the towel pack, are now produced and widely used as alternatives. Sterilized goods exposed to the air do not remain sterile and proper arrangements for packaging, storage and handling of sterilized items are an essential part of the process.

Autoclaving is the preferred sterilization option because it is highly effective, non-corrosive and, unlike chemical processes, no toxic residues are left on processed items. There are few disadvantages provided that the items withstand processing temperatures and moisture, equipment is properly maintained, steam quality is good and that staff are suitably protected from heat.

Dry heat: hot air oven

Dry heat is less efficient in destroying micro-organisms than moist heat and longer exposure times and higher temperatures are required, i.e. 160°C for 2 h, 170°C for 1 h or 180°C for 30 min (British and European Pharmacopoeias). Consequently, hot air ovens are used less frequently. They are, however, suitable for sterilizing solids and non-aqueous fluids, e.g. powders, glassware, waxes, ointments and silicone lubricants. They are also suitable for glass syringes and needles, delicate blades and other non-stainless instruments which may be blunted or damaged by moist heat sterilization.

Sterilizing ovens are electrically heated insulated boxes with perforated shelves controlled by an adjustable thermostat. A fan is fitted to circulate hot air and this ensures an even temperature throughout the processing chamber. A timer is included and the door is automatically locked on commencing the cycle to ensure items are not added or removed until sterilization is complete. Thermocouples and a chart recorder enable the user to monitor and verify that sterilizing time and temperature parameters have been met within the chamber and load. Biological indicators are not required, but chemical indicators may be used to show that the package or items have been processed. The oven should reach operating temperatures before items are added and a sufficient time given to ensure they have reached sterilization hold temperatures before timing the cycle.

Items to be hot air sterilized may be wrapped in kraft paper, tinfoil or alternatively placed in metal tubes or tins. They should then be placed on the shelving in such a way that hot air can circulate freely. Unlike autoclaving, dry heat sterilization is a lengthy process. Sterilization hold times may take up to 2 h and warm-up and cooling times more than double this. Steam sterilization is therefore the preferred option for surgical and other instruments. Items must be clean and dry before sterilization and most tolerate processing temperatures of up to 200°C.

Glass bead sterilizers are another form of dry heat sterilization. These are small electrically heated pots containing glass beads which are heated to approximately 300°C. These may be used to sterilize the cutting or piercing surfaces of instruments plunged into the glass beads. However, the process is not well controlled, items cannot be wrapped and burn incidents could occur during instrument removal or if the sterilizer is overturned.

Ethylene oxide

Ethylene oxide (EO) is widely used commercially to sterilize single use items. It is also used in some, usually the larger, hospitals for packaged reusable heat-sensitive devices (Babb *et al.*, 1982). EO is extremely penetrative, non-corrosive and, if correctly used, highly effective as a sterilizing agent. Unfortunately it is explosive, flammable, toxic, mutagenic and potentially carcinogenic and it has therefore to be used with extreme caution, particularly as it is odourless at concentrations below 700 ppm. The current UK maximum exposure limit (MEL) is 10 mg m^{-3} or 5 ppm averaged over an 8 h period.

The most popular hospital sterilizers are those which operate sub-atmospherically and where the gas is provided from a single use canister

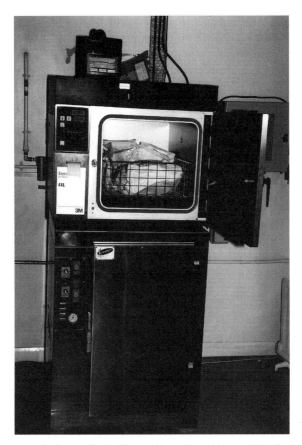

Figure 12.3   An ethylene oxide sterilizer and aeration cabinet suitable for hospital use

punctured automatically during the cycle (Figure 12.3). This reduces the likelihood of gas leaks and the subsequent toxic and explosion risks. Other machines, operating at pressures up to 5.5 bar, are available but are mainly used commercially. These utilize EO with inert gases such as fluorinated hydrocarbons, nitrogen and carbon dioxide to reduce explosion and health risks. There are other simple, non-humidified and non-controlled table top machines, but these are discouraged on safety grounds by the Department of Health and the Health and Safety Commission in the UK.

Cycle times and temperatures vary with the type of sterilizer used, but most hospital machines currently operate at 37°C or 50–55°C with total cycle times of up to 6 h. Aeration is essential for all items sterilized by EO. The duration varies and is dependent upon the absorbency of the load and the temperature and the air exchange rate of the aeration facility. If higher aeration temperatures are used, e.g. 55°C, 12 h is usually sufficient, but periods of up to 1 week of aeration may be necessary at room temperature for highly absorbent items such as PVC and rubber.

The physical and chemical parameters of the EO cycles, i.e. temperature, pressure, humidity, time and gas concentration, vary with the type of sterilizer and the nature of the load. These parameters should be monitored and checked for compliance with the manufacturers' design specification and initial performance tests. Biological indicators comprising *Bacillus subtilis* var *niger* (NCTC 10073) spores dried onto suitable carriers and contained within the load, chamber or testpieces, e.g. Line and Pickerill Helix, are necessary for cycle validation.

Ethylene oxide sterilization is most suited to large sterile service departments where trained staff and a dedicated area with exhaust ventilation is available for the sterilizer and aeration equipment. Heat-sensitive items most suited to the process include flexible fibreoptic endoscopes, electrical equipment, cardiac catheters, prosthetic devices and ophthalmic instruments.

A typical EO sterilization cycle includes: air removal with a vacuum pump, heating to the required operating temperature, usually 37°C or 55°C, steam humidification of the load to attain a relative humidity of 60%, exposure to EO for the specified sterilizing period, gas removal, air flush and finally aeration to elute residual EO from the load. Ethylene oxide should never be used where a steam sterilization option is available. It is inappropriate for soiled items, particularly those coated with oil, blood or other organic materials. Processed items may be wrapped, provided that the material is permeable to EO. The preferred wrapping materials are spun-bonded polyolefin (Tyvek) or polyethylene/paper peel packs. Advice on EO sterilization can be found in HTM 2010 (NHS Estates, 1994/95); the *Guidance on Decontamination* (Medical Devices Agency, 1993/96); and the Working Part Report on the decontamination of heat-labile equipment (Central Sterilizing Club, 1986).

Low-temperature steam and formaldehyde

Low-temperature, or sub-atmospheric steam and formaldehyde (LTSF) is a combined moist heat and chemical sterilization process (Alder, 1987; Hurrell, 1987). Formaldehyde has been used as a fumigant for many years, but is a slow sporicide and insufficiently penetrative for narrow-lumened devices. However, when used with dry saturated steam produced sub-atmospherically, it becomes a far more effective sterilant and is used as an alternative process to EO for sterilizing heat-sensitive items in some hospitals.

Instruments and equipment most suitable for processing include rigid endoscopes, particularly those used for minimal access surgery which may be damaged if repeatedly autoclaved, and devices manufactured from rubber, plastics and other heat-labile materials. Items should be clean, accessible to steam and formaldehyde and able to withstand processing temperatures of 73–80°C.

LTSF sterilizers are complicated and expensive and consequently require regular and skilled maintenance. Formaldehyde is toxic, irritant, possibly mutagenic and should be handled with extreme caution. A trained operator is required and, in the UK, care taken to ensure that the exposure limit of 2.5 mg m^{-3} (2 ppm) is not exceeded. A typical cycle would include air removal by evacuation and the introduction of formaldehyde (produced by evaporating formalin) and entrainment in sub-atmospheric steam at 73°C. The exact nature of the cycle varies with the sterilizer manufacturer, but most introduce the formaldehyde to steam in a series of sub-atmospheric pulses. The quantity of formaldehyde used, the depth of the vacuum and the holding time also vary.

After sterilization, formaldehyde is removed with a series of sub-atmospheric steam pulses, a vacuum pulled to dry the load and filtered air is admitted to return the chamber pressure to atmospheric so that the load can be removed. As the cycle parameters vary with the machine it is necessary to monitor the process microbiologically in addition to recording physical data such as time, temperature and pressure. *Bacillus stearothermophilus* spores, dried onto carriers and produced to an appropriate specification, are used to commission the machine and monitor each cycle. These may be placed in the chamber-free space, packaged items or in a testpiece such as the Line and Pickerill Helix. Formaldehyde-sensitive paper is available which may be used to assess the penetration and distribution of formaldehyde vapour. Details of this process and performance testing can be found in HTM 2010, the Medical Devices Agency *Guidance on Decontamination* and the CSC Working Party Report on the decontamination of heat-labile equipment, as cited earlier.

Low-temperature steam and formaldehyde is preferred to EO because it is a much safer process. Escaping formaldehyde has a distinctive odour and can be detected at concentrations well below the current exposure limit. Also, unlike EO, it is not flammable or explosive and is rarely absorbed into processed items. Lengthy aeration is therefore unnecessary. Unfortunately a number of problems have been encountered by those using this process, e.g. a failure to sterilize due to poor penetration, gas layering, condensation and a difficulty in obtaining suitable biological indicators. Lengthy incubation periods are required to establish the sporicidal lethality of the process. These problems, and the introduction of washer disinfectors which combine the processes of cleaning and disinfection, have reduced confidence in this as a decontamination process. However, with or without formaldehyde, sub-atmospheric steam is a highly effective method of disinfection and is preferred to immersion in disinfectants (see Chapter 11).

Gas plasma

Another sterilization option recently introduced for heat-sensitive medical devices is the use of gas plasma. This process is claimed to have overcome many of the safety concerns associated with EO and LTSF sterilization, and process times are much shorter.

Gas plasma is a highly excited body of gas produced by the application of energy to gas under vacuum. The ions and molecules within the plasma collide to produce free radicals which are capable of interacting with micro-organisms to disrupt their function. This principle has been used to develop a number of systems for sterilizing heat-sensitive instruments and other medical devices. The most well known of these systems is the Sterrad™ sterilizer from Advanced Sterilization Products, Irvine, California. This system utilizes a low-temperature (< 50°C) hydrogen peroxide gas plasma (Jacobs and Kowatsch, 1993; Crow, 1995).

The Sterrad™ process is initiated by pulling a vacuum to remove air and water. A small volume of concentrated hydrogen peroxide in aqueous solution is then injected from a cassette. This is vaporized and dispersed throughout the chamber and load. A further reduction in pressure is then applied and an electric field created using radio waves. This generates a gas plasma from the hydrogen peroxide. The free radicals produced react with and destroy micro-organisms present on precleaned, dry accessible surfaces. This procedure is repeated and, in the final stage of the process, the sterilization chamber is returned to atmospheric pressure by the introduction of filtered air. On completion of the cycle a printout is produced with the date, cycle number, stages, pressures, time, etc. The gas plasma process has advantages over EO and LTSF, as the process times, i.e. 50–80 min, are much shorter, aeration is unnecessary and no toxic emissions or residues are said to result from the process. There are, however, some drawbacks. Lumened devices, such as rigid and flexible endoscopes, can only be processed if special adapters are used to introduce the sterilant to the lumen. The system is unsuitable for very long-narrow lumened devices, particularly those closed at one end. This includes the Line and Pickerill Helix testpiece used to validate EO and LTSF sterilization processes. Hydrogen peroxide is absorbed by certain materials preventing the normal pressure changes during a cycle and causing it to abort, e.g. materials containing cellulose, instruments that have bisphenol and epoxy coatings or components made of polysulphones or polyurethane. Other requirements are that only compatible packaging can be used and items must be thoroughly clean and dry otherwise the cycle will abort. Wrapping materials made of low absorbers such as polypropylene are most suitable. Nylon- and cellulose-containing materials are incompatible.

As with other low-temperature sterilization technologies, bacterial spores, e.g. *Bacillus subtilis* and *B. stearothermophilus*, are necessary for process validation. These are dried onto suitable carriers and placed in the chamber or incorporated into packs or testpieces.

The Sterrad™ process is new and this and other gas plasma sterilization technologies are still undergoing development and scrutiny in many countries. Those considering purchasing a gas plasma system are advised to check load suitability and compatibility first. Gas plasma as a sterilization process is not yet included in the UK's Medical Devices Agency (DoH) decontamination guidelines as a sterilization option, but has been evaluated (Kyri *et al.*, 1995) and is being used in some UK hospitals.

Sporicidal disinfectants

Some disinfectants (sterilants) are capable of destroying bacterial spores in addition to vegetative bacteria, fungi and viruses. These may be used at ambient or elevated temperatures for sterilizing heat-sensitive items at their point of use. The selection and use of disinfectants were discussed in Chapter 9, but a summary of the properties of sporicidal disinfectants is included here.

The most widely used sporicidal disinfectant for instruments is 2% glutaraldehyde. It is effective against viruses, fungi, bacteria and spores. It is also non-damaging to metals, plastics, rubber, lens cements and other instrument components. It is therefore particularly suitable for processing flexible or other heat-sensitive endoscopes (Ayliffe *et al.*, 1992; Babb, 1993). Unfortunately it is toxic, irritant and sensitizing, and precautions should be taken to avoid skin and eye contact and vapour inhalation. It is also a relatively slow sporicide (Babb *et al.*, 1980) and immersions of 3–10 h have been recommended to meet stringent test requirements (i.e. destruction of 10^6 chemically tolerant spores). It is therefore a far less rapid and less effective process than sterilization using steam. In practice, much shorter exposures of 10 min to 1 h are adopted (high-level disinfection) for invasive items, as there is usually insufficient instruments and time for longer immersions. Also, the probability of there being large numbers of pathogenic spores present after thorough cleansing is most unlikely. Other disinfectants with good sporicidal activity include: the chlorine-releasing agents, i.e. sodium hypochlorite or sodium dichloroisocyanurate, at high concentrations, i.e. >1000 ppm av Cl; peracetic acid 0.35% and 0.2% (NuCidex, Steris) and chlorine dioxide (Tristel, Dexit and Medicide) (Babb *et al.*, 1980; Bradley *et al.*, 1995; Babb and Bradley, 1995). These products, when freshly prepared, kill spores in under 10 min. However, they are usually more expensive and less stable than glutaraldehyde. They are also more damaging to instruments and processing equipment, although they are claimed to incorporate corrosion inhibitors to lessen this effect. Peracetic acid and chlorine/chlorine dioxide are probably safer to use than glutaraldehyde, but they are also listed as irritant and care should be taken to prevent inhalation, skin and eye contact.

The problem with all disinfectants is that to ensure satisfactory performance items should be thoroughly cleaned first, totally immersed to exclude entrapped air and rinsed afterwards to remove toxic residues. Recontamination after processing is likely, as drying is often difficult and items cannot be wrapped to protect them from the environment. Sterile (autoclaved) or filtered water < 0.45 μm should be used for rinsing all invasive items.

Disinfectants should never be used for instruments and equipment which can more easily and safely be disinfected or sterilized using hot water or steam. Modern rigid endoscopes, many of which are used for minimally invasive surgery, are autoclavable and this method of processing is preferred to immersion in chemicals (see Chapter 11). Also, endoscope accessories and other items which are difficult to process in-house may be purchased pre-sterilized as single use items.

Other methods of sterilization

Irradiation is an industrial process and is particularly suited to the sterilization of large batches of similar heat-sensitive packaged items. Sterilization is achieved using gamma rays or accelerated electrons. A dose in excess of 25 kGy (2.5 mrad) is accepted as providing adequate assurance of sterility. Irradiation is not a process suited to hospitals, although many of the single-use heat-sensitive items purchased by health care establishments have been processed by this method. It is unsuitable for re-sterilization as this may lead to structural deterioration of the device.

Filtration, unlike other methods of sterilization, does not involve killing organisms but their removal. It is particularly useful for fluids and gases including air. Micro-organisms and particles are removed by passage through fibrous and granular depth filters or the more popular synthetic membrane filters. Micro-organisms are either trapped on the surface or within the filter. They are useful for sterilizing heat-sensitive solutions, organic solvents and oils. Many filters are autoclavable. Those of 0.2 μm or 0.45 μm should retain bacteria. Pre-filters, of larger pore size, should be used to prevent the blocking of bacteria-retaining filters. Fluids sterilized in this way should be collected into a sealed, sterilizable container. Filtered (bacteria-free) tap water is currently popular for rinsing endoscopes to remove toxic disinfectant residues before instruments are reused.

Transmissible spongiform encephalopathies

The Advisory Committees on Dangerous Pathogens (ACDP) and Spongiform Encephalopathies (SEAC) have jointly prepared (1998) guidelines on safe working practices and the prevention of infection with transmissible spongiform encephalopathy agents (TSEs). TSEs are caused by infectious proteins currently referred to as prions (see page 25).

Prions exhibit an unusual resistance to conventional physical and chemical decontamination methods (Taylor, 1992). They are not significantly affected by the disinfectants normally used for instruments, environmental surfaces, tissue or the skin. They are also resistant to gaseous sterilants, including ethylene oxide and formaldehyde, to ionizing, ultraviolet and microwave radiation and to autoclaving using conventional times and temperatures, i.e. 121°C for 15 min and 134°C for 3 min. The advice given by ACDP, SEAC and the Medical Devices Agency is that instruments that have been used on patients with known or suspected Creutzfeldt–Jakob disease or related disorders, and 'at-risk' patients where they have been exposed to brain, spinal cord and eye tissue, must be disposed of by incineration. Instruments used on at-risk patients where there has been no involvement of the brain, spinal cord or eyes should be thoroughly cleaned, preferably using an automated system, and sterilized or disinfected using an appropriate physical or chemical process. The few processes that are currently identified as suitable are:

- porous load steam sterilization at 134–137°C for a single cycle of 18 min (or 6 successive cycles of 3 min each, although this may not be completely effective);*or*
- immersion in sodium hypochlorite, 20 000 ppm av cl for 1 h;*or*
- immersion in 2 mol l^{-1} sodium hydroxide for 1 h (also not known to be completely effective)
- formic acid at 96% for 1 h – recommended for histological samples.

These chemical agents at the concentrations and contact times specified may have a detrimental effect on clinical instruments and equipment and should only be used after seeking advice from the manufacturer to ensure that the device will withstand these corrosive processes.

References

Advisory Committee on Dangerous Pathogens and Spongiform Encephalopathy Advisory Committee (1998) *Transmissible Spongiform Encephalopathy Agents: Safe Working and the Prevention of Infection*, London, HMSO.

Alder, V.G. (1987) The formaldehyde/low temperature steam sterilizing procedure. *J. Hosp. Infect.*, **9**, 194–200.

Ayliffe, G.A.J., Coates, D. and Hoffman, P.N. (1984) *Chemical Disinfection in Hospitals*, London, Public Health Laboratory Service.

Ayliffe, G.A.J., Babb, J.R. and Bradley, C.R. (1992) Sterilization of arthroscopes and laparoscopes. *J. Hosp. Infect.*, **22**, 265–269.

Babb, J.R. (1993) Disinfection and sterilization of endoscopes. *Curr. Opin. Infect. Dis.*, **6**, 532–537.

Babb, J.R. and Bradley, C.R. (1995) A review of glutaraldehyde alternatives. *Br. J. Theatre Nurs.*, **5**, 20–24.

Babb, J.R., Bradley, C.R. and Ayliffe, G.A.J. (1980) Sporicidal activity of glutaraldehydes and hypochlorites and other factors influencing their selection for the treatment of medical equipment. *J. Hosp. Infect.*, **1**, 63.

Babb, J.R., Phelps, M., Downes, J. *et al.* (1982) Evaluation of an ethylene oxide sterilizer. *J. Hosp. Infect.*, **3**, 385.

Bradley, C.R, Babb, J.R and Ayliffe, G.A.J. (1995) Evaluation of Steris System 1 peracetic acid endoscope processor. *J. Hosp. Infect.*, **29**, 143–151.

British Dental Association (1996) *Infection Control in Dentistry*, London, British Dental Association.

British Medical Association (1989) *A Code of Practice for Sterilization of Instruments and Control of Cross Infection*, London, British Medical Association.

British Standards Institution (1990) *Sterilizing and Disinfecting Equipment for Medical Products, BS 3970 Part 1: Specification for General Requirements; Part 3: Specification for Sterilizers for Wrapped Goods and Porous Loads; Part 4: Specification for Transportable Steam Sterilizers for Unwrapped Instruments and Utensils*, London, British Standards Institution.

Central Sterilizing Club (1986) Sterilization and Disinfection of Heat Labile Equipment. Working Party Report No. 2. Obtainable from the Hospital Infection Research Laboratory,

Crow, S. (1995) Gas plasma sterilization – application of space-age technology. *Infect. Control Hosp. Epidemiology.*, **16**, 483–487.

Hurrell, D.J. (1987) Low temperature steam and formaldehyde (LTSF) sterilization. Its effectiveness and merits. *J. Sterile Manage.*, **5**, 40.

Jacobs, P. and Kowatsch, R. (1993) Sterrad sterilization system: a new technology for instrument sterilization. *End. Surg.*, **1**, 57–58.

Kelsey, J.C. (1972) The myth of surgical sterility. *Lancet*, **2**, 1301.

Kyri, M.S., Holton, J. and Ridgway, G.L. (1995) Assessment of the efficacy of a low temperature hydrogen gas plasma sterilization system. *J. Hosp. Infect.*, **31**, 275–284.

Medical Devices Agency (1993/96) *Sterilization, Disinfection and Cleaning of Medical equipment: Guidance on Decontamination. Part 1: Principles; Part 2: Protocols; and Part 3: Procedures* (in preparation), London, HMSO.

Medical Devices Agency (1997) *The Purchase, Operation and Maintenance of Bench Top Steam Sterilizers*, Device Bulletin MDA DB 9605, London, Department of Health.

NHS Estates (1994/95) *Sterilization*, Health Technical Memorandum 2010, London, HMSO.

Taylor, D.M. (1992) Inactivation of unconventional agents of the transmissible degenerative encephalopathies. In *Disinfection, Preservation and Sterilization*, 2nd edn (A.D. Russell, W.B. Hugo and G.A.J. Ayliffe, eds), Oxford, Blackwell, pp. 171–179.

13

Laundering

Hospital linen and clothing should be laundered between patients, if it becomes visibly soiled, or at least weekly. The laundry process should remove evidence of previous use, including organisms, even though the risk of surviving organisms causing infection in a subsequent user is small. Laundry items are not sterile, since small numbers of microbes will be deposited on them from the air and during handling.

Although no standards are available and routine microbiological testing is unnecessary, the following guidelines may be helpful if there is a problem with the process. The average mean microbial count from the surface of used hospital linen is between 10 and 20 organisms/cm^2 when sampled with contact plates (25 cm^2). These consist predominantly of Gram-negative bacilli (about 50%), skin organisms and aerobic spore-bearing bacilli. After washing and drying and before despatch, the majority of organisms are likely to be coagulase-negative Gram-positive cocci in small numbers. The number of organisms should be reduced to approximately 1/cm^2 or fewer on sampling with a contact plate (Collins *et al.*, 1987). The presence of larger numbers of Gram-negative bacilli or *Bacillus* spp. spores after washing suggests that recontamination has occurred during the later stages of the process, e.g. from presses or recirculated water. It may also indicate inadequate drying. High counts of *Staph. aureus* or enterococci are suggestive of inadequate heat disinfection. Other more accurate methods of determining bacterial contamination have been described, but usually involve destruction of the item to be tested (Barrie, 1994). Laundering is not a sterilization process and cannot be expected to kill bacterial spores, although in practice they are not usually present in large numbers. However, rare outbreaks of infection have been associated with linen contaminated with large numbers of *Bacillus cereus*. These include meningitis following neurosurgery and umbilical infections in a neonatal unit (Barrie *et al.*, 1992).

Handling of hospital linen (see general notes on handling contaminated hospital waste, Chapter 15)

Used linen should be removed from the patient or bed with care. Unnecessary agitation of fabrics can markedly increase the number of bacteria in the air.

It is possible, though not very likely, that a single fibre shed from the linen of the patient with a staphylococcal infection may contain sufficient bacteria to initiate an infection if it settles on a susceptible wound. However, these particles are quite large and will resettle rapidly. It is preferable that susceptible wounds are not exposed within 15 min of bed making, although this is not always possible. Used linen should not be counted or sorted in the patient environment, and even when enclosed in a bag and properly closed it should not be handled roughly, dropped or kicked, as this may force contaminated aerosols or particles into the ward air.

Failure to remove foreign objects, particularly if metal or sharp, e.g. needles or scissors, from used linen can cause extensive and very expensive damage to laundry machinery or injure and infect sorting personnel. This is particularly important for categories of linen enclosed in water-soluble bags or bags with water-soluble membranes which will be placed in machines unopened. If this problem could be eliminated and sorting avoided, categorizing would be unnecessary and all linen (apart from heat-labile) could be treated in the same way.

Any used linen, which includes both soiled and fouled, may be contaminated with potential pathogens. The risk of these organisms infecting a healthy person is small if reasonable care is taken even when items are visibly fouled, provided they are handled with care (Taylor, 1982). The most important measures to prevent transfer of infections are careful handling of the linen, i.e. with gloves, and good handwashing after handling. 'Infected' linen should be sealed as soon as possible in a bag which is impervious to microbes. If water is able to penetrate the surface of the bag, it is probable it will also enable microbes to pass through the bag. Laundry bags should, therefore, not be stored in wet places and must be protected during transport.

The category of linen inside a laundry container should be clearly indicated on the outside. The following colour coding is taken from the NHS Executive (1995) guidelines, HSG (95) 18:

- *'Used'* (soiled and foul): a white or off-white bag
- *'Infected'*: a red bag or with a red prominent feature on a white or off-white background. Additionally, the container should carry a bold legend on a prominent yellow label, such as 'Infected linen'.
- *Heat-labile*: a white bag with a prominent orange stripe.

Disinfection and categories of laundry

Wherever possible all used hospital laundry should be heat disinfected in the washing process and although there are occasional failures, disinfection is usually completed in the drying and pressing stages (Figure 13.1).

Temperature requirements

All hospital linen capable of withstanding the required temperature should be best disinfected during a wash cycle, preferably by heat. There is no international consensus on temperatures required to disinfect linen and often temperatures in excess of 90°C for 10–20 min are recommended. Some

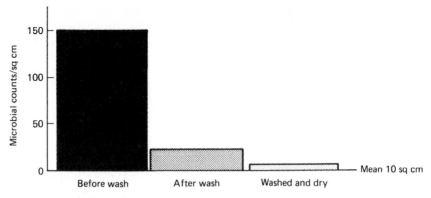

Figure 13.1   Microbial count in hospital linen (contact plates). Gram-negative bacilli were still
detectable after washing, but not after drying and pressing

countries recommend chemical disinfection as a routine. Recommendations
in the UK are based on tests with enterococci, which are more resistant to
heat than most vegetative organisms and viruses and are as follows: the
temperature of the cycle should reach a minimum of 65°C for not less than
10 min or preferably 71°C or more for not less than 3 min. These temperatures
must be reached and maintained in the coolest part of the load. A sufficient
preheating time must be allowed for the required temperature to be reached.
The time required will vary with the machine and the load, but at least
5 min will usually be required. Most vegetative bacteria and viruses, including
HIV, are heat-sensitive and should be readily killed at 71°C for 3 min.
Although the minimal temperature required to kill HBV is unknown, the
combined washing and heat processing should render the linen safe. Strains
of enterococci surviving these recommended temperatures and exposure
times have been described (see Chapter 3), but should not be a problem if
the linen is well washed and dried (Wilcox and Jones, 1995); 80°C for
1–3 min is more effective (Bradley and Fraise, 1996). However, there is no
clinical indication for changing the present recommendations, but ICTs may
wish to modify these depending on the local situation. Higher temperatures
for longer times are more costly and may damage the fabric. Removal of
blood and secretions is the essential part of the decontamination process.

Spores, e.g. *Clostridium difficile* and *Bacillus cereus*, will not be killed by
these temperatures, but sterilization of laundry would not be cost effective
and is unnecessary. Numbers are considerably reduced by rinsing in
uncontaminated water. Good maintenance and cleaning of machines and
water storage tanks will reduce the likelihood of heavy contamination with
Bacillus spores or Gram-negative bacilli.

Washing machines should be tested on commissioning to ensure standards
of disinfection are reached. They should have heat sensors which measure
the temperature of the load and these should be tested at regular intervals
as part of a quality-control programme. Routine microbiological monitoring
should be unnecessary, but may be required during an outbreak or for a
particular microbiological problem.

Categories of linen

Earlier DHSS guidelines HM(71)49, recommended that linen should be divided into two main categories:

1. Foul or 'infected': consisting of items visibly soiled with human excretions or secretions, or known to have been in contact with a patient suffering from a range of specified infections.
2. Soiled: consisting of all other used linen.

Foul or 'infected' items were to be contained in a water-soluble bag and placed directly into the washing machine without sorting. This has caused problems. Considerable sorting was required at ward level, the cost of soluble bags was often high, since in some units, such as elderly care, the majority of linen was classified as foul or infected. Machines were damaged by sharp items accidently included in unsorted loads. Heat-sensitive fabrics were not removed and therefore damaged by the heat disinfection cycle. For these reasons some managers considered it necessary to sort foul or 'infected' linen. This meant that linen that had been in contact with patients with specific infections, possibly transmissible by this route, was inadvertently handled since it was not separately identified. Although the risk of transmission was small it was felt to be unacceptable.

The present guidance recommends sorting in the ward and departments into three categories (NHS Executive (1995)):

1. *Used* (soiled and foul): all linen not covered by other named categories, irrespective of its state. Local policy may prefer not to sort foul linen and the category of foul and infected may be retained. Water-soluble bags or bags with a water-soluble seam are recommended for heavily fouled linen. It was common practice for laundries to have a central disinfection area or barrier for separating foul and infected from clean linen. While this is no longer considered necessary on the grounds of preventing infection, it may be a contractual requirement, particularly if the laundry also processes non-hospital linen. A dedicated washer–extractor machine for infected linen, in which the effluent from the drain is sealed, is still required in the UK guidelines.
2. *'Infected' linen.* The term 'infected', meaning linen from an infected patient as defined below, is an inappropriate term for linen potentially contaminated with certain pathogens. However, it is convenient and easily understood by laundry staff and is probably preferable to the alternatives 'infectious' or 'contaminated'. The 'infected' linen category contains linen from patients with or suspected of having enteric fever or other salmonella infections, dysentery, hepatitis A, B or C and carriers of these viruses, open pulmonary tuberculosis, HIV infection, notifiable diseases and other infections in hazard groups 3 and 4 (Department of Health, 1990) and also other infections specified by the Infection Control Doctor as hazardous to staff. Although it is recognized that linen which is not fouled or blood-stained from these patients is probably of low risk and that any linen may be contaminated from unknown carriers, it would seem rational to separate this group, unless sorting can be eliminated for all linen and the contents transferred to a washing

machine without handling. However, linen from most notifiable diseases is not hazardous and could be treated in the usual manner. Linen from MRSA-positive patients is not hazardous to laundry staff, but some Infection Control Teams may prefer to treat it as infected linen to avoid cross-contamination of clean linen, although there is no evidence that this is a hazard in a well-organized laundry. Linen in the 'infected' category should be sealed in a water-soluble bag at the point of use and then placed in an outer bag. The outer bag should be impervious and colour coded as described above. This bag should be washed at the same time as the contents. The water-soluble bag should be placed unopened in a machine known to have an efficient heat disinfection cycle. Linen potentially contaminated with organisms in hazard group 4 was previously recommended to be steam sterilized before laundering, but is now included with other infected linen. However, the decision should be based on the individual organism.

3.   *Heat-labile*: this includes fabrics likely to be damaged by the temperature required for thermal disinfection. Where these would otherwise have been categorized as 'infected' they will require chemical disinfection. A chlorine-releasing compound is added to the penultimate rinse to give a final concentration of 150 ppm av Cl. Chlorine-releasing compounds should not be used on fabrics treated for fire retardance. Alternative agents more suitable for use in washing machines are required for laundry disinfection, but further research is required, e.g. hydrogen peroxide, paracetic acid and quaternary ammonium compounds.

The necessity for the present UK classification remains uncertain. There is no evidence that linen from isolation units has more microbial contamination than other hospital linen or that double bagging is necessary (McDonald and Pugliese, 1996). Since universal precautions (e.g. gloves, aprons) are recommended for initial segregation of linen by ward staff, sorting of all linen could be carried out by laundry staff using similar precautions (see below), as in the USA. However, it could be argued that it would be less hazardous to transfer heavily contaminated linen, e.g. from a patient with dysentery or a salmonella infection, directly into a washing machine without sorting. Elimination of the need to sort would still be preferable and should be the objective.

Risk to laundry workers

The risk of acquisition of infection from linen by laundry workers appears to be very low, although prospective studies have not been made.

Fouled linen, unless from patients with known or suspected gastrointestinal infection, is likely to be contaminated with the same organisms as other used linen though they may be present in greater numbers. These organisms usually consist of the normal faecal flora and are unlikely to cause infections in healthy laundry workers, providing care is taken.

Protective clothing should be provided for those handling used linen prior to the disinfection stage. This should include good-quality rubber gloves, overalls, a plastic apron and, where required, waterproof boots. The laundry worker should not leave the laundry in potentially contaminated clothing and preferably it should not be possible to enter or leave the area where used linen is handled without passing through a room provided with at least a wash hand-basin. The provision of shower and changing facilities is also recommended. It is essential that workers handling used linen before the disinfection stage are taught the importance of washing their hands before leaving the work area as well as the benefit of wearing the protective clothing provided.

On employment, staff should be tuberculin or Heaf tested or should be able to demonstrate evidence of a successful BCG vaccination. If tuberculin negative, BCG should be offered. Immunization against poliomyelitis and tetanus should be offered. Typhoid vaccination is of uncertain value, and is rarely advised.

The risk of transfer of hepatitis B and C viruses to laundry workers from the linen itself is remote, provided that hygienic precautions are taken. However, there is a possibility that sharp objects, such as hollow-bore needles, may have been inadvertently left among the linen, and these could be hazardous to laundry workers. Hepatitis B vaccination is desirable.

Tunnel or continuous batch washers

Tunnel or continuous batch washers are increasingly being used in laundries. However, recontamination of the finished product may occur and is more likely to occur if recycled water is used. Organisms tend to grow overnight while the machine is not in operation, and it is recommended that the machine is run until empty and then heat disinfected before restarting. It is recommended by the NHS Executive that these machines are not used for infected linen. Pre-wash sections cannot be thermally disinfected as a routine and there is a potential for blockage, requiring maintenance staff to enter a potentially contaminated machine. 'Infected' linen, therefore, should be washed and disinfected in a washer extractor machine kept for this purpose. However, the use of washer extractors in addition to continuous batch machines can be expensive. These repairs would seem to be infrequent and appropriate protective clothing is available for engineers. The use of continuous batch washers for all laundry, including infected, should be possible.

Domestic washing machines in small units

Domestic-type washing machines are increasingly used in small units or because it is felt that the hospital laundry damages personal clothing, such as knitted items. These machines may be acceptable where those using the clothing are reasonably healthy, but not for infected or immunocompromised patients unless appropriate temperatures can be reached or chemical disinfection can be incorporated in the cycle. However, dilution during the washing process will remove most organisms. It is particularly important that the clothing is thoroughly dried after washing. If there is any doubt a microbiological check of the finished product may be useful. If the total count on a contact plate is not more than 1 organism/cm^2, the process is probably acceptable. It is advised that a laundry process with a heat disinfection cycle is used during outbreaks of infection. As the potential hazard is dependent on the type of infection, advice should be obtained from Infection Control Staff.

Nurses' uniforms and working clothing of other staff in contact with patients, linen or clinical waste are often taken home for washing. There is little evidence of spread of infection by this route. However, it is undesirable, particularly if contaminated with body fluids. If it is necessary to take clothing home for washing, it should be enclosed in a plastic bag, washed separately and thoroughly dried.

The use of commercial laundries

Where hospital laundering is contracted to an outside laundry, hospital policy relating to disinfection should be followed and steps should be taken to ensure that the proposed process will adequately disinfect. Measures considered necessary to protect hospital staff when handling used linen should also apply to non-hospital staff handling the same type of material and this should include appropriate immunization. A member of the ICT should provide advice to the management on contracts and should preferably visit the laundry to assesss hygienic compliance before awarding the contract. Periodic hygienic inspection is advised, e.g. annually.

Summary

Hospital linen should not be an infection risk to subsequent users. Processing should be monitored and a documented quality-control system introduced. A Hazard Analysis Critical Control Points (HACCP) method could be usefully be used (see Chapter 14, page 182). Temperatures and exposure times, treatment of rinse water, if potentially contaminated, in-use chlorine concentrations, and drying temperatures, are all examples of critical points. Microbiological tests may be useful for initial validation or during outbreaks, but should not be required as a routine.

References

Barrie, D. (1994) How hospital linen and laundry services are provided. *J. Hosp. Infect.*, **27**, 219–235.

Barrie, D., Wilson, J.A., Hoffman, P.N. and Kramer, J.M. (1992) *Bacillus cereus* meningitis in two neurosurgical patients: an investigation into the source of the organism. *J. Infect.*, **25**, 291–297.

Bradley, C.R. and Fraise, A.P. (1996) Heat and chemical resistance of enterococci. *J. Hosp. Infect.*, **34**, 191–196.

Collins, B.J., Cripps, N. and Spooner, A. (1987) Controlling microbial contamination levels. *Laundry Clean. News*, 30–31.

Department of Health Advisory Committee on Dangerous Pathogens (1990) *Categorization According to Hazard and Categories of Containment*, London, HMSO.

McDonald, L.L. and Pugliese, G. (1996) Laundry service. In *Hospital Epidemiology and Infection Control* (C.G. Mayhall, Ed), Baltimore, Williams & Wilkins.

NHS Executive (1995) *Hospital Laundry Arrangements For Used and Infected Linen* (HSG (95) 18), Heywood, Lancs, Health Publications Unit.

Taylor, L.J. (1982) Is it necessary to treat foul linen from geriatric patients as infected? *J. Hosp. Infect.*, **3,** 209–210.

Wilcox, M.H. and Jones, B.L. (1995) Enterococci and hospital laundry. *Lancet*, **344,** 594.

14

Catering

The hospitalized patient is more susceptible to food-borne infection and more likely to suffer serious consequence from such infection than healthy members of the community. It is difficult to compare the risk of food-borne infection related to hospitals with the risk from food prepared elsewhere. Not only will a high proportion of hospital patients be more susceptible but the chance of food-borne infection being diagnosed and recorded is very much higher in the hospitalized patient. The tendency to centralize food preparation in hospitals also means that a single lapse in food hygiene can put large numbers at risk. Although the risk of an outbreak in an individual hospital is small, the highest standards must be maintained due to the susceptible population.

Most countries have similar legislation on food safety. In the UK, food safety law is now mainly based on the Food Safety Act 1990 and the Food Safety Regulations, 1995. These regulations were updated in accordance with the European Community Council Directive 93/43/EEC (1993). The main requirements are included in the Health Service Guidelines (1996). The Food Safety (Temperature Control) Regulations, 1995 recommend a lower storage temperature of 8°C or less and a higher storage temperature of 63°C or more. Although these temperatures will limit the growth of food-poisoning organisms, a lower temperature should be used if possible, especially in hospital refrigerators. In this chapter, a lower storage temperature of 5°C or less is recommended as in previous guidelines.

To ensure food safety, a detailed policy concentrating on correct purchasing, handling, processing and distribution of food should be produced (Barrie, 1996). The state of repair and decoration is less relevant to the spread of infection, but the establishment should be clean and a cleaning schedule should be prepared and followed.

Training and supervision of staff is more important than occasional inspections. Although hospital catering establishments in the UK will be inspected at intervals by an Environmental Health Officer (EHO), routine inspections (e.g. 1–2 times per year) should also be made by a member of the Infection Control Team, the catering manager and a member of the estates department. The EHO and ICT should collaborate on standards required and on staff training.

The Infection Control Doctor and Nurse have an overall responsibility for assessing risks of infection in the hospital, including catering, and for advising the Chief Executive on balancing available resources for control of infection.

Hospital catering is often provided by an outside contractor. Similar standards of hygiene and staff training are required as for hospital catering staff. The ICT and the EHO should be involved in contract specification and should monitor the processes set up by the contractor.

Pest control

Cockroaches and other pests are common, particularly in old hospitals. A number of studies have demonstrated the presence of pathogens, e.g. salmonella, in cockroaches, but evidence that they are responsible for epidemics is inconclusive. Nevertheless, control and, if possible, eradication is desirable as a general hygienic measure. A trained pest control officer should be appointed to prepare and monitor pest control contracts (Baker, 1981; Department of Health, 1992).

Food poisoning

Food poisoning may occur if large numbers of specific organisms or preformed microbial toxins are ingested; for example, the infective dose of salmonella in a healthy person is about 10 000 organisms, but much smaller numbers will cause an infection in a person with absent gastric acid. These large numbers occur either because the food has not been properly cooked or the organisms have been allowed to grow unchecked in food due to storage at temperatures between 8°C and 63°C, although the majority of pathogens grow best between 15°C and 45°C. Some organisms, e.g. campylobacter, *E. coli* 0157 and viruses, can cause infection with a much lower number of organisms, and listeria can grow at temperatures below 5°C

Outbreaks of food poisoning in hospitals are mainly caused by *Salmonella* spp. or less frequently by *Clostridium perfringens* and *Staph. aureus*. Other organisms, e.g. *Bacillus cereus*, enteropathogenic or toxigenic strains of *E. coli*, *Vibrio parahaemolyticus* and enteric viruses, such as hepatitis A and the Norwalk virus. Protozoa, such as cryptosporidium and giardia, may also cause outbreaks but these are usually associated with the community. *Campylobacter* spp. are the commonest causes of infective diarrhoea, but are rarely responsible for outbreaks in hospitals. *Listeria* infections may rarely be acquired from food, mainly from dairy products, such as soft cheeses

Salmonella spp. are carried in the intestinal tracts of humans and animals and are mainly found in foods of animal origin, especially meat, poultry and eggs. The symptoms are usually diarrhoea and occasional fever, appearing 6–24 h after ingesting the food.

Clostridium perfringens is similarly a contaminant of meat and produces a toxin in the intestine after ingestion which causes diarrhoea in 8–24 h. It produces spores which may survive normal cooking processes and which will then grow if food is not stored at low temperatures after cooking.

Staphylococcus aureus is carried in the nose or on the skin of some normal individuals (see page 38) and may be transferred to food on the hands or from an infected lesion on catering staff. The staphylococci grow in food and produce a toxin which causes vomiting, usually in 1–6 h.

Bacillus cereus is a spore-forming organism and is often found in cooked rice which is not stored at low temperature after cooking. It produces a toxin both in the originally contaminated food and in the organisms subsequently growing in the intestine after ingestion. Symptoms may be rapid in onset, e.g. vomiting after 1–6 h, or delayed, e.g. diarrhoea after 8–16 h.

Escherichia coli. Enteropathogenic or toxigenic strains are responsible for traveller's diarrhoea and food poisoning. They are carried in the intestinal tract of man and animals and are likely to be introduced into the kitchen in raw meat or poultry. Most of the strains produce toxins causing diarrhoea and occasionally vomiting, 18–24 h after eating contaminated food. *E.coli* 0157:H7 produces a verotoxin which can cause a very severe, often bloodstained, diarrhoea (haemorrhagic colitis), vomiting and sometimes kidney failure requiring hospital treatment. The small number of organisms required to cause an infection increases the problems of controlling an outbreak.

Campylobacter spp. are found in raw animal foods, including milk. It causes diarrhoea, abdominal pain and fever after an incubation period of 3–5 days and symptoms may continue for a week or more. Person-to-person spread is uncommon.

Mode of spread

- Hands of staff contaminated from raw or inadequately cooked meat or poultry, or from inadequately cleaned equipment and preparation surfaces.
- Hands of staff carrier of a food-poisoning organism who has not washed after defaecation.
- Directly to patients or staff in uncooked or inadequately cooked food stored at room temperature.
- Septic lesion on skin of member of staff, often on hands.

Investigation of outbreaks

Ward staff should be encouraged to report to the ICT as soon as possible if there are an unusual number of patients or staff with diarrhoea and/or vomiting. Appropriate samples should be sent to the laboratory and should include samples from infected staff before being sent off duty.

The ICN will visit the wards to determine if these are genuine infections and to collect all the necessary information. This will include the type of symptoms, time of onset and dietary history over the past 48 h. A comparison of food eaten by infected patients and non-infected controls is necessary if food poisoning is suspected. The public health medical officer (e.g. CCDC) should be informed and if necessary the ICT and EHO should examine hygienic procedures in the kitchen and take microbiological specimens if appropriate. Some hospitals may save samples of food for this purpose, but this is rarely a cost-effective procedure.

Faecal carriers of the outbreak strain in the catering staff are often victims rather than causes of the outbreak.

Cases occurring at the same time in several wards suggest food poisoning, although small numbers throughout the hospital may reflect an outbreak in the community rather than spread in the hospital. A slowly spreading infection with the number of cases building up over some days is rarely caused by food poisoning but by person-to-person spread.

If the outbreak is caused by an organism which may spread from person to person, e.g. salmonella, control of infection measures will be required. These are not required if the outbreak is due to a toxin-producing organism which does not spread, e.g. *Cl. perfringens* and *Staph aureus*.

Depending on the number of cases and their severity, the Infection Control Doctor must decide in consultation with the CCDC whether the major outbreaks committee should be convened.

Prevention of infection

Adequate cooking

Destruction of micro-organisms depends on exposure of the food to an adequate temperature for a defined time. Most cooking procedures should destroy vegetative bacteria if the process is well controlled. Heat penetrates dense masses slowly and minimal temperatures may be found in the coldest part of the load, e.g. the centre of the thickest part of a joint of meat, or a container of mashed potato or milk pudding. Few cooking processes can guarantee to kill heat-resistant spores. A balance must be maintained between adequate cooking and ruining good food by excessive heat. Measurement of the temperature of food during cooking or at the end of the cooking period is rarely carried out and the more frequent use of a suitable thermometer with an appropriate probe for sampling the internal temperature of food masses is recommended (Figure 14.1). The centre of the food should reach 70°C

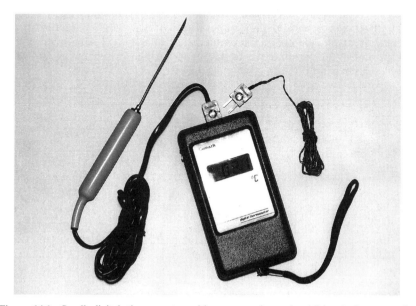

Figure 14.1 Small digital thermometer with meat probe and additional thermocouple. Recommended for checking the temperature of food and processing equipment

for 2 min or 80°C for 1 min or other equivalant time/temperature relationship. The presence of unaltered haemoglobin, in the fluid or meat, suggests that temperatures above 60°C have not been reached. In one test, the internal temperature of a joint of beef described by the chef as 'well done' did not exceed 42°C during the process. Rare (undercooked) beef is preferred by many people and rarely causes harm but it can be responsible for outbreaks of infection and should not be given to hospital patients. Undercooked poultry or pork is never acceptable. The use of carefully defined menus, which include the maximum size of joints and minimum cooking temperatures and times, is strongly recommended. Policies for the reuse of food prepared for other purposes and the length of time which food, once prepared, can be stored before discarding should be included.

Cooking times are usually based on the whole process starting at room temperature, and inadequate defrosting of frozen products can lead to substantial and hazardous undercooking. Once adequately cooked, the temperature of the food should be retained at above 63°C until eaten or should be chilled rapidly to 3°C (see p. 184). Reheating of cooked food should be avoided except as part of a properly planned chilled meal service. Where this is unavoidable it should be cooled rapidly and stored below 5°C until required. Large joints of meat and bulk foods may cool very slowly; the centre may remain at bacterial growth temperature for long periods, even if refrigerated. Using small joints and spreading mince, etc. out on trays will facilitate rapid cooling. Cooked foods capable of supporting bacterial growth, e.g. soups and gravies, which will be stored and reheated, should not remain out of the refrigerator for more than 2 h. No part of the food should be at a temperature of above 8°C and below 63°C for more than 4 h. Food kept at these temperatures for longer periods is not necessarily inedible or unsafe, but with good management these guidelines can be achieved in hospital practice. It must also be appreciated that when reheating food in stocks or sauces the temperature of that stock or sauce is not necessarily an indication of the temperature of the food suspended within it. Catering staff should use temperature measuring equipment regularly and particularly when adopting new procedures.

Salad vegetables and fruit

Salad vegetables served uncooked should always be examined carefully and well washed under running water before being served. They are frequently heavily contaminated with a wide range of Gram-negative bacilli including *E. coli, Ps. aeruginosa* and *Klebsiella* spp. While these organisms can be ingested in large numbers by healthy people without causing harm, they can cause invasive infections in the heavily immunosuppressed patients, such as those being treated for leukaemia, and it may be necessary to serve only cooked food to such patients. The skin of fruit may also be contaminated and should be washed and dried. It is preferable to remove the skin immediately before the fruit is eaten by the very susceptible patient.

Segregation of cooked and uncooked food

Raw meat and poultry, fresh fish and raw vegetables should all be assumed to be contaminated with potential food poisoning organisms. Separate preparation areas, each with their own equipment and staff, should ideally be provided. Although fish can be prepared in the meat bay, there is a risk of transferring the distinctive odour and taste of the raw fish to the meat. Plastic aprons are usually worn for preparing these foods. These aprons should be removed and the hands thoroughly washed and dried by staff before handling any food that will be eaten without further heat treatment. If implements or other materials which have been in contact with raw meat, fish, poultry or raw vegetables have to be used for other purposes, they must be properly washed and thoroughly dried before reuse.

Storage

Any food which contains moisture should be stored at temperatures below 8°C or preferably below 5°C. This will prevent the multiplication of most bacteria, but will not kill existing bacteria. There are certain obvious exceptions, such as raw fruit and vegetables, which may be stored for short periods without refrigeration. Although most food poisoning organisms are unlikely to grow below 5°C, bacterial enzymes which cause food spoilage may remain active. Deep-freezing at $-18°C$ will inhibit most enzymes but will not kill bacteria. Ward refrigerators should be checked daily and should be run at temperatures of not more than 5–7°C.

Food preparation surfaces, crockery and cutlery

Detailed schedules defining methods, materials and frequency of cleaning for each item should be produced and displayed in each department. The schedules should define who is responsible for carrying out each task and supervision should be based on the written schedules. While it is probable that fluctuation in demand or absence of staff will make it difficult to maintain schedules on occasions, clearly indicated priorities will ensure that essential work is carried out.

Food preparation surfaces should be clean and dry before use. The commonest cause of heavily contaminated food preparation surfaces is recent cleaning with a contaminated cloth and failure to allow sufficient time for the surface to dry thoroughly. While it is recommended that stainless steel or other impermeable surfaces are used this is less important than good cleaning and thorough drying, preferably using a disposable paper wipe or clean dry cloth. If a good technique is used, disinfection is rarely needed and is never a substitute for good hygiene.

Crockery and cutlery washed in a machine with a final rinse temperature of 80°C or above for 1 or more minutes, and allowed to dry before use, should be microbiologically safe. This is more efficient than washing by hand even with a detergent/disinfectant solution (Table 14.1). Washing by

Table 14.1 Bacterial counts from washed plates		
Method	No. sampled	Counts of 10 or more per contact plate (25 cm²)
Hand-washed	108	68 (63%)
Machine-washed	72	5 (7%)

hand should preferably be carried out in a double sink with a final rinse in clean hot water. Visibly moist crockery or cutlery should not be used but disinfection may not be required except rarely after use by infected patients, or during outbreaks. Disinfectants are never required if adequate temperatures are reached during the washing and rinsing processes. Disposable crockery is sometimes provided for use by patients with a communicable disease, but is not usually necessary.

Handwashing

It is necessary to instruct food handlers specifically when, where and how to wash their hands. Studies have shown that even well-trained nurses can miss vital areas such as tips of fingers or thumbs when not properly instructed (see Figure 6.1). A wash-basin reserved exclusively for handwashing, with a designated person responsible for ensuring that soap and paper towels are always available, should be provided at each work bay. It is difficult to persuade caterers (or any other staff) to walk more then a few feet to wash their hands. Poorly sited wash-basins are not used. Washing with soap and water is generally adequate and disinfectants are unnecessary unless recommended by the ICT, e.g. during outbreaks. All food handlers should receive some basic training in food and personal hygiene. Disposable gloves should preferably be worn when handling food to be eaten without further heating, e.g. sandwiches.

General comments

Equipment which is intended to keep food at a controlled temperature, either hot or cold, should be checked regularly and wherever practical a clearly visible thermometer should be incorporated as part of the equipment. A daily inspection by a supervisor or manager to ensure that equipment is operating at the right temperature and that storage policy, e.g. separation, and stock rotation is understood and carried out as recommended.

Complaints of undercooking or of keeping hot food below the required temperature should be investigated thoroughly. Failure to maintain standards on one occasion could result in a disastrous outbreak.

Heated food trolleys are intended to keep hot food warm and not to heat food. Hot food must, therefore, be at a temperature of 63°C or above when placed in the trolley. A period of approximately 30 min should be allowed for the trolleys to reach the required temperature before use and they must be kept on until food service is completed. The ability of the trolley to maintain food at the appropriate temperature can deteriorate and should be checked at regular intervals (monthly).

Hazard Analysis Critical Control Points (HACCP)

To ensure safety of food and catering processes, the hospital is advised to set up a HACCP system (Richards *et al.*, 1993; Barrie, 1996). This is a structured system of identification, assessment and control of microbiological or other hazards in the production, processing, preparation, storage and distribution of food.

- Hazards are likely to be associated with conditions which allow potential pathogens to grow in food, e.g. failure to heat food sufficiently and failure to store food at a temperature which will prevent growth of micro-organisms.
- A critical point is a point in an operation at which control can be exercised to eliminate, prevent or minimize a hazard. Examples include temperature of food after cooking, recording of time spent at room temperature after cooking, recording of refrigerator temperatures and time taken for food to reach this temperature. These control points should be related to bacterial survival and growth under the conditions of the system in use.
- The process should be defined by means of a flow chart, identifying the hazards, both microbiological and toxic. It should include raw materials, the processes involved, e.g. times and temperatures of cooking, chilling and refrigeration, characteristics of ingredients, quality assurance, management systems, details of shelf life and handling by customer. From this initial exercise, it should be possible to identify the hazards and critical control points and to introduce monitoring and verification procedures. It is also necessary to ensure that the system is able to detect rapidly and correct any failures in the monitoring procedures.

Summary of important control measures

- Good separation of naturally contaminated food from food already cooked or likely to be eaten without cooking.
- Adequate cooking to destroy food-poisoning organisms and heat-labile toxins.
- Storage at a temperature likely to prevent the growth of food-poisoning organisms, e.g. less than 5°C (8°C or less, legal requirement) or above 63°C.
- High standards of catering and personal hygiene promoted by adequate training and enforced by constant supervision.

Faecal screening

Outbreaks are rarely due to faecal carriers on the staff and even if routine tests are made this does not guarantee that all carriers will be identified or that epidemics are less likely. Screening gives a false sense of security. Hygiene standards should be high enough to ensure that food is not contaminated with faecal organisms. Screening policies are often irrational; carriers may excrete only very rarely, perhaps once a year. If staff were screened before employment, annually or even every 6 months, they may well become infected the next day, or be missed. Screening for typhoid carriers may be a justifiable precaution in countries, or in staff from countries, where typhoid is common. Carriers may be difficult to treat effectively and any sudden introduction of a screening programme may well mean the loss of staff who, despite their carriage, have worked safely and efficiently for many years.

Much larger numbers of enteric pathogens may be excreted immediately after an infection than in a chronic carrier even though symptoms have disappeared, and it is essential that catering staff are trained and actively encouraged to report any incident of diarrhoea or vomiting in themselves or their families. They are, however, unlikely to be co-operative if temporary absence from the normal duties leads to loss of pay.

Pre-cooked chilled foods

There has been a rapid expansion in the use of pre-cooked chilled meals in hospitals. In this system food is cooked, packed, rapidly chilled and stored refrigerated for up to 5 days before being portioned and distributed. The food is then reheated (regenerated) in purpose-built equipment immediately prior to consumption. The advantage of this system is that it enables the work load of kitchens to be spread over a longer period, reducing peak demands at meal times. It should also provide a greater variety of menu, but does lead to increasing centralization. The centralization of food preparation services and increased storage time involved could be expected to increase the risk of food-borne infection. In practice the degree of control and monitoring built into pre-cooked chill systems, usually absent from traditional catering systems, adequately compensates for the increased risk. There has as yet been no outbreak of food-borne infection associated with cook-chilled foods in hospital. Careful examination of working systems has, however, shown that with some practices there can be an unacceptable increase in the level of organisms present (Wilkinson *et al.*, 1991).

New systems require detailed planning well in advance of implementation (see HACCP system, page 182). A flow chart of the proposed system should be prepared from the arrival of the food on site to the final point of consumption. Each stage should be examined for potential infection risks. The correct work flow patterns and the permissible time and temperature range for each type of food passing through an area should be agreed. Monitoring systems to ensure that the accepted parameters are not exceeded should also be set up and the relevant documentation prepared. A clear chain of command and responsibility should also be established. Any readings taken, e.g. temperatures, must be reviewed by a manager who will accept responsibility for taking action or not doing so. Changes may have to be made in the light of operational experience, but systems should be in place before operations commence. The Department of Health (1989) guidelines on precooked chilled foods should be used as a basis for drawing up operational systems. The basic requirements of these guidelines is that following cooking (70°C for at least 2 min), food should be reduced to a temperature of 3°C within 90 min and then stored at a temperature of 3°C for not longer than 5 days, including the day of preparation and the day of consumption.

Regeneration should occur within 30 min of removal from chilled storage and the food heated to 70°C for at least 2 min and served within 15 min of reheating.

If during storage the temperature of the food rises to 5°C it must be consumed within 12 h and if it rises to 10°C it should be discarded. These guidelines do, however, include substantial safety margins and over-rigorous interpretation can erode potential cost savings without reducing infection risks and can adversely affect the acceptability of the food served. Consultation with the Environmental Health Officer at an early stage is advised but it is important to differentiate between advice given as a legal requirement and personal preference of the officer giving it. Requirements should be clearly backed by law or should be a clearly demonstrable risk that can be backed with microbiological evidence or case histories. The CCDC should be asked to differentiate and provide evidence if necessary. Where it is decided that departure from the guidelines is necessary the reason for doing so should be recorded and the process should be monitored microbiologically until it is considered safe. The records should be kept permanently. Any problem should be referred to the Infection Control Doctor. The microbiologically quality of the food should be at an acceptable level prior to regeneration and regeneration temperatures should not be relied on to render it safe. Not all foods are equally suitable for this process, though this may depend on the method of regeneration. Some gravies and sauces may separate and skinned and sliced meat can dry out. Dishes with a high moisture content, such as casseroles, may be most suitable but it cannot be assumed that traditional dishes can necessarily be prepared by this method. Regular monitoring of the temperature of the regenerated food is required. Monitoring should not always be from the same point or the same trolley, since failure of a single heating plate in the trolley can occur unnoticed. Each trolley should be marked so that tests are carried out in rotation and all points are tested over a given period.

Microbiological testing may be necessary at the initial stages to ensure that all systems are working consistently and to a reliable standard. However, when the physical parameters necessary to ensure this have been established, microbiological monitoring can be stopped unless further investigation is necessary. Recording thermometers on all refrigeration plants are recommended.

Some organisms may survive or even multiply at the temperatures used for storing chilled food, e.g. *Listeria* spp. The risk from such organisms can, however, be exaggerated. They tend to occur in a limited range of products, including goat's cheese and commercially prepared salads. These products are often kept at low temperatures for very long periods and are unlikely to be part of a hospital diet. However, a careful watch is required for potential pathogens that may grow at low temperatures, since there are increasing reports of food poisoning by these organisms.

References and further reading

Baker, L. (1981) Pests in hospitals. *J. Hosp. Infect.*, **2,** 5–9.
Barrie, D. (1996) The provision of food and catering services in hospital. *J. Hosp. Infect.*, **33,** 13–33.

Department of Health (1989) *Chilled and Frozen. Guidelines on Cook-Chill and Cook-Freeze Catering Systems*, London, HMSO.

Department of Health NHS Management Executive (1992) *Pest Control Management*, HSG(92)35, London, HMSO.

Food Safety Act (1990) London, HMSO.

Food Safety (Temperature Control) Regulations (1995) London, HMSO.

Health Service Guidelines, NHS Executive (1996) *Management of Food Hygiene and Food Services in the National Health Service*, HSG(96)20, London, HMSO.

Hobbs, B.C. and Roberts, D. (1993) *Food Poisoning and Food Hygiene*, 6th edn, London, Arnold.

Richards, J., Parr, E. and Riseborough, P. (1993) Hospital food hygiene: The application of Hazard Analysis Critical Control Points to conventional hospital catering. *J. Hosp. Infect.*, **24,** 273–282.

Wilkinson, P.J., Dart, S.P. and Hadlington, C.J. (1991) Cook-chill, cook-freeze, cook-hold, sous vide: risks for hospital patients? *J. Hosp. Infect.*, **18** (suppl. A), 222–229.

15

Clinical waste disposal

Waste is being produced in increasing amounts throughout the world and disposal is becoming more difficult and expensive. Landfill sites are now less readily available and environmentally safe incinerators are expensive and if not well maintained can produce toxic emissions.

Clinical waste disposal is more expensive than domestic and should be kept to a minimum. Unnecessary costs of disposal of clinical waste diverts funds from patient care. Every effort should be made to use reusable medical equipment and to recycle as much waste as possible (Daschner and Dettenkofer, 1997).

Categories of waste

Hospital waste is classified into two main categories: household and clinical/medical or, more recently, health care risk waste. Definitions of clinical waste vary in different countries, but usually refer to materials which are potentially hazardous and associated with patient or animal diagnosis or treatment and medical research.

Clinical waste is mainly dealt with here as a potential infectious hazard, but may include toxic agents, such as dangerous drugs and radioactive materials.

● Domestic and clinical waste are both likely to contain moisture and nutrients which will allow micro-organisms, especially Gram-negative bacilli, to grow to large numbers on storage in the environment. These micro-organisms, e.g. *Pseudomonas aeruginosa*, found in both domestic and clinical waste are opportunistic pathogens, i.e. can cause infection in susceptible subjects, particularly in hospital. Several studies have shown that fewer organisms are usually present in clinical waste and potential pathogens are often of similar types, e.g. salmonella and HIV, to those in domestic waste (see Hedrick, 1989; Ayliffe, 1994).

● Most human pathogens which spread from person to person survive poorly on storage in the environment at room temperature and even if they survive, the likelihood of their causing an infection decreases rapidly with time spent outside the human body.

- There is little evidence of acquisition of infection in handlers of domestic or clinical waste, although needle stick injuries have caused infections in clinical and nursing staff and intravenous drug users.

In view of these findings, it would seem reasonable to consider the classification of clinical waste. The risks to handling staff from clinical waste depend on the likelihood of relevant micro-organisms in waste causing an infection (Hedrick, 1989).

Requirements for infection to be transmitted

- The presence in the waste of a pathogen of sufficient virulence or in sufficient numbers to cause an infection.
- A mode of transfer to the host, e.g. the hands.
- A portal of entry into the host, e.g. the mouth or an operation site.
- A susceptible host, e.g. with an exposed traumatic wound.

On the basis of these requirements, a risk assessment can be made; for example, a surgical dressing contaminated with blood from a patient infected with a bloodborne virus is unlikely to cause an infection in a waste handler wearing gloves and taking reasonable hygienic precautions. Sealing the dressing in an impermeable plastic bag will remove the risk.

Health care workers in clinical areas are at a greater risk as they are responsible for initial handling, segregation and containment of the waste, and needle stick injuries are one of the greatest hazards, but even these are relatively low risk (see page 46).

The risk of HIV infection from contamination of a mucous membrane with HIV-contaminated blood is only 0.09% and even a needle stick injury from an HIV-contaminated needle only causes 0.25% infections. Nevertheless, in view of the severity of the infection and absence of a definite cure with treatment, excessive precautions tend to be taken. The risk of acquiring HCV from a contaminated needle is uncertain, but probably low, e.g. 1–2%. The risk of acquiring HBV from a contaminated needle is higher, e.g. 20%, but health care staff and all handling clinical waste should be immunized.

Wound dressings, incontinence pads, stoma bags and babies diapers are frequently heavily contaminated by the normal flora of the intestinal tract and skin and could be disposed of as domestic waste, as is usually the case in the community of most countries (Ayliffe, 1994). There is obviously room for considerable savings by reducing the amount of clinical waste.

Based on the above assessment of infection risk, a collaborative document on infectious waste disposal produced by 13 societies involved in the management of infections in the USA has suggested three categories of infectious waste (Regulated Medical Waste, 1993):

- sharp instruments (used and unused)
- laboratory microbiological cultures and other microbiological waste
- selected waste from highly infectious human and animal sources, i.e. infections caused by risk category 4 organisms.

Some may also prefer to include waste from other infected patients, e.g. typhoid and open tuberculosis, in this category.

Human tissues are low risk, but are perceived by the public as potentially hazardous and are aesthetically unacceptable. They are usually treated as clinical waste and incinerated.

Legal aspects of waste disposal

In most countries, there is considerable legislation on waste disposal, but it tends to be general and not usually too prescriptive. The UK is influenced by European Union Directives which are likely to increase legal requirements in the future (Moritz, 1995). Clinical waste is defined in the UK Controlled Waste Regulations, 1992. These state the following. Clinical waste consists of:

1. Any waste which consists wholly or partly of human or animal tissue, blood or other body fluids, excretions, drugs or other pharmaceutical products, swabs or dressings, or syringes, needles or other sharp instruments, being waste which *unless rendered safe* may prove hazardous to persons coming into contact with it.
2. Any waste arising from medical, nursing, dental, veterinary, pharmaceutical or similar practice, investigation, treatment, care, teaching or research, or the collection of blood from transfusion, being waste which *may cause infection* in any person coming into contact with it.

These regulations are broad and do not indicate the detailed requirements to meet them. The Environmental Protection Act 1990 and the Duty of Care Regulations, 1991 require a 'Duty of Care' on 'any person who imports, produces, carries, keeps, treats or disposes of controlled waste, or as a broker, has control of such waste to take all such measures applicable to him in that capacity as are reasonable in the circumstances to prevent the escape of waste from his control or that of another person' (Moritz, 1995). The 'Duty of Care' under the Act means that the responsibility of the hospital authorities extends not only from outlying areas to a central site within the hospital, but also to ensure that waste is suitably contained and labelled for transport outside the hospital and that the carrier is an authorized person. Failures to comply can result in criminal prosecution.

Prosecutions can also be brought in the UK under the Health and Safety at Work Act 1974 and the Control of Substances Hazardous to Health Act Act (COSHH, 1988).

Guidance based on current regulations and produced by the Health and Safety Commission (Health and Safety Commission Services Advisory Committee (HSAC), 1992), or an appropriate modification of this guidance is usually accepted as a requirement. Clinical waste is classified by the HSAC as follows:

- *Group A.* All human tissues, including blood (whether infected or not), animal carcasses and tissues from veterinary centres, hospitals and laboratories, and all related swabs and dressings. Waste materials, where the assessment indicates a risk arising from, for example, infectious disease cases. Soiled surgical dressings, swabs and other soiled waste from treatment areas.

- *Group B*. Discarded syringe needles, cartridges, broken glass, and any other contaminated disposable sharp instruments or items.
- *Group C*. Microbiological cultures, and potentially infected waste from pathology departments (laboratory and post-mortem rooms) and other clinical or research laboratories.
- *Group D*. Certain pharmaceutical products and chemical wastes.
- *Group E*. Items used to dispose of urine, faeces and other bodily secretions or excretions assessed as not falling in Group A. These include used disposable bedpans or bedpan liners, incontinence pads, stoma bags and urine containers.

Groups A, B and C are required to be incinerated. Incineration is preferred for Group E, but certain secure landfill sites would be acceptable.

Although these guidelines are frequently used as a basis for prosecution, they are not legally enforceable and, as already discussed, many of the items included can scientifically be demonstrated as low risk to the individual and to the environment, especially in Group E. It is illogical to include items commonly used in the community (e.g. babies diapers, stoma bags, incontinence pads or occasional wound dressings) as clinical waste.This causes problems with elderly patients and is not cost effective. However, requirements for waste disposal have to take into consideration aesthetic apppearances and public perception of hazard as well as scientific risk. Variations in practice from that recommended should be discussed with the regulating authorities. Some of these items in bulk can be offensive and require special disposal arrangements.

General management of clinical waste

A hospital should have a waste strategy and should be able to demonstrate it has a safe disposal system. A waste disposal officer should be appointed and there should be a written policy. This should include removal of spillage, e.g. if a waste container breaks during transport, wearing of protective clothing, covering all lesions with an impermeable dressing and ensuring that staff handling waste are immunized against tetanus and hepatitis B. The waste disposal officer should liaise with relevant departments, e.g. supplies and services and occupational health (HSAC, 1992).

A hospital waste management committee, consisting of the waste disposal officer, infection control staff, a pharmacist, a Health and Safety officer, representatives of medical and nursing staff and a risk manager, if available, may be useful.

Training programmes should be provided for relevant staff and these should be updated and audited at intervals.

The policy should be realistic and followed by staff, as it could be used in a court of law as evidence, although it should be recognized that occasional errors, especially in segregation, occur in most hospitals without creating any infection problem.

The most important part of the disposal system is initial segregation of waste at source. Poor segregation can be very costly to a hospital in terms of an unecessary amount of clinical waste.

Clinical waste should be sealed in a strong impermeable plastic bag of a defined colour, e.g. yellow in the UK, and labelled with place and date of origin. Bags should be removed regularly, e.g. twice daily, from clinical areas, and kept in safe and secure storage. Domestic waste should be contained in a bag of a different colour, e.g. black in the UK.

The producer of clinical waste has to ensure that waste is transferred to an authorized person and that there is a written description of the waste.

Sharps disposal

All needles and sharp instruments for disposal should be discarded into a sharps container which is resistant to penetration by sharp instruments and fluids. Specifications are available in many countries, e.g. BS 7320 (1997), Health and Safety (SI), 2095, (1996), in the UK. Containers should not be overfilled, i.e. not more than two thirds full, and should be kept out of reach of children.

The opening in the container for sharps should not also allow removal of contents.

Storage of containers should be secure, and handling should be minimal, since penetration by sharps can occur in certain unusual circumstances.

Human tissue

Where there is a need to dispose of identifiable human tissue, e.g. limbs and placentae, it should be enclosed in a clinical waste bag, labelled and transported immediately to an incinerator under the supervision of a responsible person and placed directly in the incinerator.

If it is necessary to transport tissues outside of the hospital, the yellow bag should preferably be placed in a rigid locked container which contains the name and telephone number of a responsible person in the hospital. Although the tissues are unlikely to be a hazard to the public, their appearance in a road following an accident could cause offence and undue adverse publicity.

Laboratory waste

All cultures and patient specimens for discard should be autoclaved on site if possible, before final disposal in clinical waste bags, although there is no scientific reason why effectively autoclaved waste should not be disposed of as domestic waste. In the UK, it is contained in a light blue bag or clear bag with blue lettering.

If autoclaving is not possible in the hospital laboratory, the waste should be transferred as clinical waste for incineration, preferably but not necessarily on site.

Other methods of treating clinical waste

The costs and problems of incineration, particularly in individual hospitals, have led to the use of other methods of waste decontamination (Blenkharn, 1995; Collins and Kennedy, 1993). These include steaming, maceration, microwaving, plastic densification and chemical disinfection, e.g. using chlorine-releasing compounds or paracetic acid. Some studies have shown that microwaving is effective and might be appropriate in certain circumstances, but whether any of these methods will be accepted or considered necessary for general use is uncertain.

The escalating costs of commercial waste disposal may require rethinking by hospital authorities in the future. A smaller incinerator could become cost effective if used with other measures. Other methods, such as microwaving, might be less expensive than incineration if the waste could subsequently be disposed of as domestic waste. Disinfection would be adequate and sterilization is not required. Recycling as much as possible and energy redistribution associated with incineration would all reduce waste disposal costs and improve the environment.

Storage sites

These should be properly planned, sited to avoid offence, secure from people and vermin and should be cleanable. Poorly maintained sites attract vermin which may open bags and distribute contents. Although damage to bags may not represent a major infection hazard, it is clearly undesirable. It is advisable that containers for domestic and clinical waste should be segregated in hospital storage areas to avoid errors by waste collectors. Vehicles used for transport of waste to a central storage area in the hospital should preferably be used for this purpose only. If this is not possible, the inside of the vehicle should be cleaned before being used for other purposes. Waste bags should be transported in appropriate closed containers in the vehicle.

References and further reading

Ayliffe, G.A.J. (1994) Clinical waste: how dangerous is it? *Curr. Opin. Infect. Dis.*, **7**, 499–502.

Blenkharn, J.I. (1995) The disposal of clinical wastes. *J. Hosp. Infect.*, **30** (suppl.), 514–520.

Collins, C.H. and Kennedy, D.A. (1993) *Handbook No. 13.The Treatment and Disposal of Clinical Waste*. Leeds, H. and H. Consultants.

Daschner, F.D. and Dettenkofer, M. (1997) Protecting the patient and the environment – new aspects and challenges in hospital infection central. *J. Hosp. Infect.*, **36**, 7–15.

Health and Safety SI 2095, (1996) Carriage of dangerous goods. London, HMSO.

Hedrick, E.R. (1989) Infectious waste management: Will science prevail? *Infect. Cont. Hosp. Epidemiol*, **9**, 488–490.

HSAC (1992) *The Safe Disposal of Clinical Waste*, Health and Safety Commission Services Advisory Committee, London, HMSO.

London Waste Regulation Authority (1994) *Guidelines for the Segregation, Handling, Transport and Disposal of Clinical Waste*, 2nd edn. London, London Waste Regulation Authority.

Moritz, J.M. (1995) Current leglislation covering clinical waste. *J. Hosp. Infect.*, **30** (suppl.), 521–530.

Regulated Medical Waste, Definition and Treatment: A Collaborative Document, (1993) *AORN L*, **58**, 110–114.

16

Special units

Hospital sterile services department

The function of a sterile services department (SSD) is to supply a range of sterile items to theatres, wards and other departments and sometimes to the community. Dressings and other soft packs may be made up of items or materials which are purchased sterile or unsterile or prepared in the department. The department will also clean, disinfect or sterilize equipment for reuse, e.g. theatre instruments. SSDs should operate whenever possible according to the Guide to Good Manufacturing Practice (GMP). Departments are being increasingly influenced by requirements of European Directives and Standards (e.g. Medical Devices Directives EEC 93/94). If SSDs process medical devices for Health Authorities other than their own, they are required to comply with the same European Standards as are commercial manufacturers. To minimize the risk of transfer of infection from 'sterilized' items, rigorous attention must be paid to the control of the cleaning and sterilization processes. The frequency and methods of testing are described in detail in HTM 2030, (1997) (see also Chapters 11 and 12). Environmental control in other areas, e.g. for preparation of items prior to sterilization, can be excessive leading to unnecessarily frequent cleaning of surfaces and the provision of filtered air at positive pressure. Such procedures can substantially increase costs. There is no evidence of infection caused by inadequate environmental control when items have been subsequently sterilized effectively although pyrogens in fluids may be a problem.

It is important that standards are assessed in terms of infection risks and on scientific evidence. Bioburdens are likely to be much higher if cleaning of equipment is inadequate than they are from airborne contamination. Nevertheless, clean conditions are important in packaging areas and some mechanical ventilation may be required to maintain controlled conditions. Sterile items correctly packaged and stored should remain impermeable to micro-organisms. A specific shelf life is not required, provided that the packs remain undamaged and dry. A good stock rotation should ensure that packs are not stored for too long. It is also important to ensure that insects, such as Pharaoh's ants, and rodents are excluded from the sterile store or storage sites in the hospital (Baker 1981).

The SSD may also include a hospital disinfection unit (HDU). The function of this unit is to reprocess permanent medical equipment for reuse. This will usually involve cleaning, disinfection and checking that the equipment is functioning correctly. To ensure that equipment is functioning after cleaning and disinfection, it may be necessary to consult the biomedical engineering department, as specialized test equipment and additional skills may be required. It is, therefore, preferable that the two departments are in close proximity. The increasing use of minimal access surgery will increase the need for specialized processing. This would preferably be in the SSD, but an area in the theatre suite may sometimes be preferred. The processing in either area should where possible be the responsibility of trained SSD staff.

Hospital staff have become increasingly concerned with the risk of acquiring infection, especially HBV, HCV and HIV (see Chapter 3). Risk can be reduced by wearing gloves when handling blood-stained items and taking particular care when handling used, sharp instruments. Known high-risk equipment should be decontaminated at the earliest possible stage after being brought into the SSD. All instruments, etc., that require washing should preferably be heat disinfected at this stage. This is preferable to using chemical disinfectants which may themselves be a toxic hazard, or autoclaving instruments prior to washing. Autoclaving adds an additional stage and is likely to coagulate protein, making it difficult to remove at the wash stage. Heat disinfection at the wash stage may also be advantageous for some anaesthetic equipment since it should then be possible to pack it on removal from the washer without any further procedures.

However, if washer/disinfectors are to be used for either of these purposes, an improvement in standards of control is required. Agreement on acceptable cycles and methods of commissioning and regular checking of machines is necessary. The coolest part of the most difficult load would need to reach a temperature of 90°C or be raised to 80°C and held for 1 min or to 71°C for 3 min. These correspond to standards accepted for laundering. Cleaning efficiency should also be checked. It is recommended by the Department of Health that certificates are issued stating that equipment returned for servicing or repair is microbiologically safe (see Chapter 11). This may be difficult and it is advisable to state that it has been put through an effective decontamination process, if this is possible. Failed medical devices may have to be returned to the manufacturer without dismantling, and decontamination of internal surfaces may not be possible. A statement should be made to this effect, with advice on safety precautions, e.g.:

- wearing protective clothing – gloves, plastic aprons and goggles if splashing is likely
- handwashing after removal of gloves or after handling the equipment
- disinfection of the equipment after cleaning – where possible a washer disinfector should be used preferably using heat
- if equipment is heat labile, immersion in a chemical disinfectant may be required (see Chapter 11).

All external surfaces of the equipment should be cleaned before sending to the manufacturer. Although all equipment should be handled safely, the manufacturer should be informed if the equipment was used on a patient with a known transmissible infection, e.g. HIV or tuberculosis. Additional instructions from the microbiologist may be required.

Intensive care and special care baby units

The incidence of infection is usually higher in the ICU than in other wards and departments. The patients are particularly susceptible to infection and undergo a range of invasive procedures (Sproat and Inglis, 1992). The occasional requirement for an immediate response to a deteriorating clinical situation may be associated with a failure in good aseptic techniques.

The main infections are of the lower respiratory tract in patients under-going mechanical ventilation, but urinary tract infection and infections of intravascular catheter sites are common and often associated with bacteraemia (see Chapter 5). Most infections are endogenous, although patients are often colonized with an antibiotic-resistant strain before a clinical infection caused by this strain becomes manifest. The infections are mainly due to Gram-negative bacilli, e.g. *Klebsiella* spp., *Pseudomonas aeruginosa, Serratia marcescens, Enterobacter* spp. and *Acinetobacter* spp. as well as *Staphylococcus aureus*, coagulase-negative staphylococci, enterococci, *Candida* and *Aspergillus* spp. MRSA is a particular hazard (see page 56).

The architectural design has little influence on the infection rate and the dry environment, e.g. walls, floors and ceilings do not require any particular attention (Huebner *et al.*, 1989). At least one single-bedded ventilated cubicle suitable for source or protective isolation is advised if the unit has an open plan layout. Beds should be as far apart as possible (e.g. over 2 m), so that large droplets from the respiratory tract of one patient do not reach the adjacent patients, as well as allowing sufficient room for equipment and attention by staff. The direction of the airflow in the isolation room should be regularly checked. A positive pressure instead of a negative pressure could disseminate organisms throughout the unit. The site where extracted air is discharged to the outside should be chosen with care. Air extracted from an isolation cubicle entering an open window has probably been responsible for the spread of MRSA (Cotterill *et al.*, 1996). A plenum (positive pressure) ventilation system is not required to prevent the spread of infection in the main unit (Bauer *et al.*, 1990), but may be necessary to provide a suitable working environment; 8–12 air changes per hour should be sufficient. Wash-basins should be conveniently placed for staff attending any patient and should be well designed (see Chapter 8).

Medical equipment can be an important source of infection. Ease of decontamination should be considered when buying new equipment. Methods of decontamination and frequency of cleaning should be defined and preferably carried out in an equipment cleaning and disinfection department (see page 194). Static fluids or wet equipment, e.g. disinfectant solutions containing tubing, nailbrushes, mops and wet washing bowls should not be kept in the unit since Gram-negative bacilli can grow to large numbers in these. Gowns or aprons are not usually necessary unless carrying out a procedure on a patient. Masks/visors are of uncertain value, but may be worn if carrying out a suction procedure or if splashing of body fluids is likely, but not as a routine. Gloves should be worn for suction procedures and contact with blood or body fluids, for other contaminated procedures or when handling patients colonized or infected with MRSA. A separate gown or apron should be worn when attending an infected patient. Overshoes and hats are not required and adhesive or disinfectant mats at the door of the unit are of no value in reducing transmission of infection.

Handwashing is the most important technique and requires particular attention if staff move from one patient to another. Although plain soap is adequate, an antiseptic detergent, e.g. povidone-iodine or chlorhexidine, may be preferred; 60–70% ethyl or isopropyl alcohol with 1% glycerol is a rapid and effective method of hand disinfection and is particularly useful in an ICU. However, reasonable care will eliminate or considerably reduce exogenous infection but the problem of endogenous infections remains (Van Saene et al., 1991).

Similar problems apply to special care baby units. The organisms causing infection are also similar, but include infections acquired from the mother before or during delivery, e.g. Lancefield Group B streptococci, rubella, cytomegalovirus, herpes simplex, toxoplasma, HBV, HIV and many others. Group B streptococci may also be acquired by cross-infection in the unit.

Colonization of the mouth and intestinal tract with antibiotic-resistant Gram-negative bacilli is common. Infection mainly spreads from baby to baby on the hands of staff. Masks are unnecessary and individual gowns are only needed for handling infected neonates or during outbreaks. Single rooms are required for isolation of infected patients and a larger room is useful for cohort nursing. Airborne spread can occur, but is unusual, and contaminated equipment may rarely act as a common source. An antiseptic detergent preparation is usually advised for handwashing but, as in the ICU, disinfection with alcohol is particularly convenient when moving rapidly from one baby to another. Communal pots of ointments or creams should be avoided.

Incubators should be washed and dried after use by each baby; special attention should be paid to mattresses and the humidifier. Gram-negative bacilli surviving or growing on moist surfaces are the main hazards in baby incubators, and drying after cleaning is the main method of control (Ayliffe et al., 1975). Disinfection is not usually necessary, but wiping over with 70% alcohol after cleaning should be satisfactory if disinfection is required and it does not damage the incubator. Wiping over the incubator with a weak hypochlorite solution (125 ppm av cl) is also effective, but should be rinsed off with water and dried. Incubators can be conveniently cleaned in an equipment cleaning and disinfection section of the SSD.

Other items requiring regular cleaning or disinfection are suction and respiratory equipment, aerosol humidifiers, rectal thermometers, intragastric feeding equipment and baths. Infant feeds should, if possible, be sterile and expressed milk should be pasteurized and monitored bacteriologically. The pasteurizer should be regularly checked to ensure that temperatures and times are correct. In addition to pasteurization of the milk, donors of expressed breast milk should be checked for HIV antibody.

Operating theatres

The main factors associated with wound infection are considered in Chapter 5. The physical environment is of minor importance as a source of infection (Maki et al., 1982; Ayliffe, 1991a; Griethuysen et al., 1996) and frequent cleaning of walls and ceilings is unnecessary (2–4 times a year should be adequate) (Emmerson, 1992). Routine disinfection of floors is not necessary for reasons already mentioned, but if a disinfectant is used, it should be rinsed off frequently; the dried deposit (also of detergents) may affect the antistatic properties of the floor. However, antistatic floors are unnecessary if explosive anaesthetic gases are never used. Spillage should be promptly removed, and disinfected with a chlorine-releasing solution or powder if considered potentially hazardous (see Chapter 11).

A plenum ventilation system providing 20 air changes per hour should be satisfactory for general surgery and high-efficiency filters are not required. Although the filters should be as close as possible to the outlet of the ducts, this is not always possible; disinfection of ducts with formaldehyde is unnecessary. If the system is shut off overnight, the ventilation system should be run for at least 30 min before using the operating room, to remove any free particles. Measuring the air flows, exchange rates and pressure drops across doorways at regular intervals is of greater value than bacteriological sampling (see below). Smoke tests are also useful to determine air flows through doorways. The air should flow from the operating room outwards, apart from into the clean preparation room (lay-up room) which if present should have the same or slightly higher air flow as the operating room. It is important to remember that the operating room during an operation probably has more bacteria in the room than any other room in the suite, apart from changing rooms before and after operating lists.

Humidification systems should be of a steam injection type if possible, since Gram-negative bacilli will grow in most other systems, particularly if recirculation of water is involved. Nevertheless, the risk of airborne transfer of organisms from a humidifier to the theatre is small. Filters will further reduce this possibility.

Infection risks from bacteria on floors are small and there is little advantage in having a transfer area and changing trolleys, or putting on overshoes (Ayliffe et al., 1969; Lewis et al., 1990; Humphreys et al., 1991). The patient may be transferred directly from ward to operating room in a bed, provided that ward bedding is removed before entering the operating room. Adhesive or disinfectant mats should be avoided. Tests have shown that these mats do not significantly reduce the number of bacteria on the floor of the operating room (Ayliffe et al., 1967; Troare et al., 1997). If the mats are not regularly changed, anaerobic spore-bearing bacilli, e.g. Clostridium perfingens, may accumulate and could actually be transferred to shoes or trolleys.

Nevertheless, it is rational for all persons entering the clean area of the theatre to change completely into clean clothing and put on theatre shoes or boots. Although ordinary theatre clothing and cotton gowns allow bacteria to escape into the environment, most of the organisms (e.g. Staph. epidermidis and diphtheroids) are unlikely to cause infection except in implant surgery. Bacteria-impermeable clothing may be preferable for high-risk surgery. An ultra-clean air system (i.e. Charnley-type operating enclosure with a downward laminar flow system providing approximately 300 air changes per hour) is commonly used for knee and hip implant surgery. A ventilated bacteria-impermeable operating suit may be worn by the operators. This system has been shown to reduce deep infection rates when compared with conventional ventilation (Lidwell *et al.*, 1982). Effective antibiotic prophylaxis will reduce the infection rate to a similar extent, but usually the ultra-clean air system is combined with antibiotic prophylaxis.

The value of an ultra-clean air system in other types of operation is unknown, but it is unlikely to influence infection in general surgical operations. Wearing of masks does not reduce the number of airborne organisms and probably has little effect on the infection rate in general surgery (Orr, 1981; Ayliffe, 1991b; Tunevall, 1991), but again it is rational if masks are considered necessary for the operating team to wear efficient filter-type masks. Masks are now commonly worn with spectacles or goggles as a protection against blood splashes. Wearing of watches or jewellery is probably a minor infection hazard, but it is rational for the operating team to remove jewellery, apart from wedding rings. It is also rational to prevent unnecessary people entering the theatre suite, particularly the operating room, and to maintain hygienic discipline without too much ritual. Disinfection of the surgeon's hands and the operation site is also rational and has a proven bacteriological effect (Lowbury, 1992).

Although microbiological sampling of a ventilated, empty operating theatre is of doubtful value, commissioning tests are often recommended (Department of Health, HTM 2025, 1994), mainly for legal reasons. The recommendations suggest that aerobic colony counts should not exceed 35 colony-forming units per m^3 in an empty theatre. The air sampler should be operated by remote control to avoid sampling organisms released by the operator. Of greater importance than microbiological sampling is a general assessment of the theatre by the ICT and an engineer on commissioning, e.g. air flows and exchange rates (plus smoke tests), temperature and humidity, ensuring removal of builder's rubble from ducts, general cleanliness, appropriateness of wash-basins and taps and any other hygienic aspects of the environment (Holton and Ridgeway, 1993). For reasons already described (see Chapter 5), the number of organisms in the air during an operation is not usually related to the hazards of infection and routine sampling is of little value unless a specific organism is being sought during an outbreak. It is suggested (Department of Health, HTM 2025, 1994) that counts during an operation should not exceed 180 per m^3, but it is not clear how this suggested standard was obtained or its clinical relevance.

Microbiological sampling of an ultra-clean air system is more rational, since most of the air is recirculated and the organisms present are likely to cause an infection in patients with implants. A filter failure could recirculate organisms and cause an infection problem. Sampling is commonly carried out on commissioning and after maintenance. However, it is more important to ensure that the filters are working correctly by physical tests. It is suggested that air sampled at 1 m from the floor within an empty enclosure should not contain more than 0.5 colony-forming-unit per m^3.

Protective isolation units

These are commonly available for certain immunosuppressed patients, e.g. with organ transplants or leukaemia. Infections are mainly endogenous and tend to be caused by *Escherichia coli, Klebsiella* spp., *Bacteroides* spp., *Staph.*

aureus, cytomegalovirus, *Candida, Aspergillus* spp., *Pneumocystis carinii* and mycobacteria. *Pseudomonas aeruginosa* is a problem in some units.

A single room (with or without a ventilation system) is usually adequate, provided that barrier nursing procedures and techniques are good and doors are kept closed. If ventilation is required, a plenum system providing 8–12 air changes per hour should be adequate. However, the value of single room protective isolation remains doubtful (Nausef and Maki, 1981).

Masks, caps and overshoes are not usually worn. Gowns or plastic aprons are often worn and may be kept within the room for one day before changing. In some units, particularly those concerned with cardiac, liver and bone marrow transplants, precautions are often much stricter and involve full protective clothing. Laminar flow systems are now rarely used. The advantages of these complex precautions remain uncertain. There is also some evidence that oral non-absorbable antibiotics (e.g. framycetin, colistin, nystatin) help to reduce the number of infections in high-risk patients. Routine bacteriological monitoring of patients is also controversial (Daw *et al.*, 1988). The units should have suitable equipment for disinfecting cutlery and crockery and bedpans, preferably by heat. Uncooked foods, especially salads, may contain large numbers of *Pseudomonas, Klebsiella* or *Listeria* and should be avoided in high-risk patients.

General hospitals can rarely afford to staff a special protective isolation unit, but source and protective isolation patients can be nursed in the same unit provided that hygienic measures are efficient and the direction of the air flow in the cubicles can be changed as necessary (Ayliffe *et al.*, 1979; Rahman, 1985). Aspergillus infections present a special problem (see page 64).

References and further reading

Ayliffe, G.A.J. (1991a) Role of the environment in the operating suite in surgical wound infection. *Rev. Infect. Dis.*, **13** (suppl.10), S800–804.

Ayliffe, G.A.J. (1991b) Masks in surgery? *J. Hosp. Infect.*, **18**, 165–166.

Ayliffe, G.A.J., Collins, B.J., Lowbury, E.J.L. *et al.* (1967) Ward floors and other surfaces as reservoirs of hospital infection. J. Hyg. (Camb.), **65**, 515–536.

Ayliffe, G.A.J., Babb, J.R., Collins, B.J. and Lowbury, E.J.L. (1969) Transfer areas and clean zones in operating suites. *J. Hyg. (Camb.)*, **67**, 417–425.

Ayliffe, G.A.J., Collins, B.J. and Green, S. (1975) Hygiene of babies incubators. *Lancet*, **1**, 923.

Ayliffe, G.A.J., Babb, J.R., Taylor, L. *et al.* (1979) A unit for source and protective isolation in a general hospital. Br. M. J. *ed.*, **2**, 461–465.

Baker, L.F. (1981) Pests in hospitals. *J. Hosp. Infect.*, **2**, 5–9.

Bauer, T.M., Ofner, E., Just, H.M. *et al.* (1990) An epidemiological study assessing the relative importance of airborne and direct contact transmission of micro-organisms in a medical intensive care unit. *J. Hosp. Infect.*, **15**, 301–309.

Cotterill, S., Evans, R. and Fraise, A.P. (1996) An unusual source for an outbreak of methicillin-resistant *Staphylococcus aureus* on an intensive therapy unit. *J. Hosp. Infect.*, **32**, 207–216.

Daw, M.A., McMahon, E. and Keane, C.T. (1988) Surveillance cultures in the neutropenic patient. *J. Hosp. Infect.*, **12**, 251–261.

Department of Health (1994) *HTM 2025*, London, HMSO.

Emmerson, A.M. (1992) Environmental factors influencing infection. In *Infection in Surgical Practice* (E.W. Taylor, ed.), Oxford, Oxford University Press.

Griethuysen, A.J.A., van, Spies-van Rooijen, N.H. and Hoogenboom-Verdegaal, A.M.M. (1996) Surveillance of wound infections and a new theatre: unexpected lack of improvement. *J. Hosp. Infect.*, **34**, 99–106.

HBN 13, Health Building Note. Sterile Services Department (1992), NHS Estates.

Holton, J. and Ridgeway, G.L. (1993) Commissioning operating theatres. *J. Hosp. Infect.*, **23**, 153–160.

Huebner, J., Frank, U., Kappstein, I. *et al.* (1998) Influence of arcitectural design on nosocomial infections in intensive care units: a prospective 2 year analysis. *Int. Care Med.*, **15**, 179–183.

Humphreys, H. (1993) Infection control and the design of a new operating theatre suite. *J. Hosp. Infect.*, **23**, 61–70.

Humphreys, H., Marshall, R.J., Ricketts, V.E. *et al.* (1991) Theatre overshoes do not reduce operating theatre floor bacterial counts. *J. Hosp. Infect.*, **17**, 117–123.

Institute of Sterile Services Management, (1989) *Guide to Good Manufacturing Practice for National Health Service Sterile Services Departments*, London, ISSM.

Lewis, D.A., Weymont, G., Nokes, C.M. *et al.* (1990) A bacteriological study of the effect on the environment of using a one or two- trolley system in the theatre. *J. Hosp. Infect.*, **15**, 35–53.

Lidwell, O.M., Lowbury, E.J.L., Whyte, W. *et al.* (1982) Effect of ultraclean air in operating rooms on deep sepsis in the joint after operation for total hip or knee replacement: a randomised study. *Br. Med. J.*, **285**, 10–14.

Lowbury, E.J.L. (1992) Special problems in hospital antisepsis. In *Principles and Practice of Disinfection, Preservation and Sterilization* (A.D. Russell, W.B. Hugo and G.A.J. Ayliffe, eds), Oxford, Blackwell, pp. 310–329.

Maki, D.G., Alvarado, C.J., Hassemer, C.A. and Ziltz, M.A. (1982) Relation of the inanimate environment to endemic nosocomial infection. *N. Engl. J. Med.*, **307**, 1562–1566.

Mayhall, C. G. (ed.) *Hospital Epidemiology and Infection Control,* Baltimore, Williams and Wilkins.

Nausef, W.M. and Maki, D.G. (1981) A study of simple protective isolation in patients with granulocytopenia. *N. Engl. J. Med.*, **304**, 448–453.

Orr, N.W.M. (1981) Is a mask necessary in the operating theatre? *Ann. Roy. Coll. Surg.*, **63**, 390–392.

Philpott-Howard, J. and Casewell, M. (1994) *Hospital Infection Control: Policies and Procedures*, London, Saunders.

Rahman, M. (1985) Commissioning a new hospital isolation unit and assessment over five years. *J. Hosp. Infect.*, **6**, 65–70.

Sproat, L.J. and Inglis, T.J. (1992) Preventing infection in the intensive care unit. *Br. J. Int. Care*, **2**, 275–285.

Taylor, E.W. (ed.) (1992) *Infection in Surgical Practice*, Oxford, Oxford University Press.

Troare, O., Eschapasse, D. and Laveran, H. (1997) A bacteriological study of a contamination control tacky mat. *J. Hosp. Infect.*, **36**, 158–160.

Tunevall, Th. G. (1991) Postoperative wound infections and surgical masks: a controlled study. *World J. Surg.*, **15**, 383–388.

Van Saene, H.K.F., Stoutenbeek, C.P. and Hart, C.A. (1991) Selective decontamination of the digestive tract (SDD) in intensive care patients: a critical evaluation of the clinical, bacteriological and epidemiological benefits. *J. Hosp. Infect.*, **18**, 261–267.

Bibliography

Ayliffe, G.A.J. and Babb, J.R. (1995) *Pocket Reference to Hospital-acquired Infections*, London, Science Press.

Ayliffe, G.A.J., Lowbury, E.J.L., Geddes, A.M. and Williams, J.D. (1992) *Control of Hospital Infection: A Practical Handbook*, 3rd edn, London, Chapman and Hall.

Ayliffe, G.A.J., Coates, D. and Hoffman, P.N. (1993) *Chemical Disinfection in Hospitals*, 2nd edn, London, Public Health Laboratory Service.

Bartlett, C.L.R, Macrae, A.D. and Macfarlane, J.D. (1986) *Legionella Infections*, London, Arnold.

Benenson, A.S. (ed.) (1995) *Control of Communicable Diseases in Man*, 16th edn, New York, American Public Health Association.

Bennett, J.V. and Brachman, P.S. (eds). (1998) *Hospital Infections*, 4th edn, Philadelphia, Lippincott-Raven.

Caddow, P. (ed.) (1989) *Applied Microbiology*, London, Scutari Press.

Damani, N.N. (1997) *Manual of Infection Control Procedures*, London, Medical Media.

Emmerson, A.M. and Ayliffe, G.A.J. (eds) (1996) *Surveillance of Nosocomial Infections, Baillieres Clinical Infectious Diseases*, Vol. 3, No. 2, London, Bailliere Tindall.

Gardner, J.F. and Peel, M.M. (1998) *Sterilization Disinfection and Infection Control*, 3rd edn, Edinburgh, Churchill Livingstone.

Greenwood, D., Slack, R., Petherer, J. (eds) (1992) *Medical Microbiology. A Guide to Microbial Infections, Pathogenesis, Immunity, Laboratory Diagnosis and Control*, 14th edn, Edinburgh, Churchill Livingstone.

Hobbs, B.C. and Roberts, D. (1993) *Food Poisoning and Food Hygiene*, 6th edn, London, Arnold.

Infection Control Nurses' Association, London Regional Group (1995) *Infection Control Information Resources*, Harpenden, UK, Mediaprint.

International Federation of Infection Control (1995) *Education Programme for Infection Control, Basic Concepts and Training*, IFIC, 3M, UK.

Johnston, I.D.A. and Hunter, A.R. (eds.) (1984) *The Design and Utilization of Operating Theatres*, London, Arnold.

Mandell, G.L., Douglas, R.G. and Bennett, J.E. (1992) *Principles and Practice of Infectious Diseases*, 3rd edn, Edinburgh, Churchill Livingstone.

Mayhall, C.G. (ed) (1996) *Hospital Epidemiology and Infection Control*, Baltimore, Williams and Wilkins.

Meers, P., McPherson, M. and Sedgwick, J. (1997) *Infection Control in Healthcare*, Cheltenham, Stanley Thornes.

Mehtar, S. (1992) *Hospital Infection Control. Setting up a Cost Effective Programme with Minimal Resources*, Oxford, Oxford Medical Publications.

Philpott-Howard, J. and Casewell, M. (1994) *Hospital Infection Control: Policies and Practical Procedures*, London, Saunders.

Russell, A.D., Hugo, B. and Ayliffe, G.A.J. (eds) (1992) *Principles and Practice of Disinfection, Preservation and Sterilization*, 2nd edn, Oxford, Blackwell Scientific Publications.

Slade, N. and Gillespie, W.A. (1985) *The Urinary Tract and the Catheter: Infection and Other Problems*, New York, Wiley.

Taylor, E.W. (ed.) (1992) *Infection and Surgical Practice*, Oxford, Oxford Medical Publications.

Wenzel, R.P. (1997) *Prevention and Control of Nosocomial Infections*, 3rd edn, Baltimore, Williams and Wilkins.

Wilson, J. (1995) *Infection Control in Clinical Practice*, London, Bailliere Tindall.

Worsley, M.A., Ward, K.A., Parker, L., Ayliffe, G.A.J. and Sedgwick, J.A. (1990) *Infection Control: Guidelines for Nursing Care*, London, ICNA.

Index